Mechanism and
Management of Headache

Mechanism and Management of Headache

Third Edition

James W. Lance
CBE, MD, FRCP, FRACP

Chairman, Division of Neurology,
The Prince Henry and Prince of Wales Hospitals, Sydney;
Professor of Neurology,
The University of New South Wales, Sydney, Australia

BUTTERWORTHS
LONDON - BOSTON
Sydney - Wellington - Durban - Toronto

THE BUTTERWORTH GROUP

United Kingdom	Butterworth & Co (Publishers) Ltd London: 88 Kingsway, WC2B 6AB
Australia	Butterworth Pty Ltd Sydney: 586 Pacific Highway, Chatswood NSW 2067 Also at Melbourne, Adelaide and Perth
Canada	Butterworth & Co (Canada) Ltd Toronto: 2265 Midland Avenue, Scarborough, Ontario, M1P 4S1
New Zealand	Butterworths of New Zealand Ltd Wellington: T & W Young Building, 77–85 Customhouse Quay, 1, CPO Box 472
South Africa	Butterworth & Co (South Africa) (Pty) Ltd Durban: 152–154 Gale Street
USA	Butterworth (Publishers) Inc Boston: 19 Cummings Park, Woburn, Mass. 01801

First published   1969
Second edition   1973
Third edition   1978
ISBN 0 407 26457 4
© J. L. Lance 1978

British Library Cataloguing in Publication Data
Lance, James Waldo
Mechanism and management of headache – 3rd ed
1. Headache
I. Title
616.8'57   RB128   77-30545
ISBN 0 407 26457 4

Typeset by Scribe Design, Medway, Kent
Printed in Great Britain by Cox & Wyman Ltd,
    London, Fakenham and Reading

To my wife, Judith

Contents

Preface to the Third Edition

Preparation of the Third Edition has been an exacting task because of the proliferation of publications on almost every aspect of headache. With the exception of Chapters 3, 4, 5 and 13, much of the text has been rewritten. Separate chapters are now devoted to headaches thought to be caused by intracranial vasodilatation and to post-traumatic headache. The chapters on migraine have been recast to incorporate new work and to attempt to bring together present knowledge of migraine into a coherent whole. More space has been given to the psychological and physiological management of migraine and tension headache. The introduction of computerized tomography (CT scanning) has completely altered the investigation of those patients whose headaches do not fall into a typical benign pattern. The merits of each method of investigation are presented and contrasted to aid in reaching a diagnosis by the safest and most economical means. Because of the slight but inevitable expansion of the book, essential references have been cited at the end of each chapter. In spite of the bulge in its waistline, the book is still intended for having and holding and is not to be regarded respectfully at a distance.

Sydney, N.S.W.   James W. Lance

Preface to the
First Edition

About once a month, until the age of 70 years, George Bernard Shaw suffered a devastating headache which lasted for a day. One afternoon, after recovering from an attack, he was introduced to Nansen and asked the famous Arctic explorer whether he had ever discovered a headache cure.

'No,' said Nansen with a look of amazement.

'Have you ever tried to find a cure for headaches?'

'No.'

'Well, that is a most astonishing thing!' exclaimed Shaw. 'You have spent your life in trying to discover the North Pole, which nobody on earth cares tuppence about, and you have never attempted to discover a cure for the headache, which every living person is crying aloud for.'

It is easy for a person who has never been troubled with headaches to lose patience with those who are plagued by them. The reaction of the virtuous observer may pass through a phase of sympathetic concern to one of frustrated tolerance and, finally, to a mood of irritation and resentment in which the recurrence of headaches is attributed to a defective personality or escape from unpleasant life situations. The sound sleeper is traditionally intolerant of the insomniac and the speedy of bowel is just a little contemptuous of the constipated. In short, we tend to consider ourselves as the norm and to look quizzically at those whose physiological or psychological processes are at variance

*Pearson, H. (1942). *Bernard Shaw*. pp. 242–243. London: Collins

xi

with our own. Such an attitude often persists in spite of years of advanced education and scientific training. To make it clear that I am not numbering myself among the righteous, I must state that I am not subject to headache and that my spirits often sink when confronted with a succession of patients whose contorted expressions testify to a lifetime of headache misery. This is about the only circumstance which I find likely to provoke headache in myself — I suppose on the principle that, if you can't beat them, join them!

It would be foolish to deny that the workings of the mind are of great importance in the production of headache, but they are only part of the story.

My interest in migraine was first aroused when working at the Northcott Neurological Centre in Sydney. Each patient with migraine gave a history that was a little different from the others but all were variations on a clearly recognizable theme. It seemed that all the clues were there to point the way to the understanding of the mechanism of migraine. These thoughts led to studies of the clinical features and natural history of migraine and, later, to laboratory work which now suggests that migraine is an hereditary recurrent metabolic disturbance. If this be the case, a patient cannot be held responsible for having migraine attacks any more than a woman for having menstrual periods. The treatment of migraine has improved with better understanding of the syndrome but knowledge of the migraine mechanism and its treatment still leave much to be desired.

Mysteries remain in the problem of tension headache although the place of psychological factors is much more obvious in this group than in migraine and an association with chronic over-contraction of muscle is most universal. However, many tense, frowning people do not get headaches and the explanation for those that do must go beyond a catalogue of undesirable personality traits and bad luck in cards or love. Migraine and tension headache are given most space in this small book because they are common complaints, not always easy to diagnose and treat, and worry patients and their medical attendants. Other common forms of headache such as those arising from eyestrain or sinusitis are not emphasized as much, because their mechanism and management are more straightforward. Serious acute headaches which betoken some hazardous intracranial condition are described sufficiently to assist in diagnosis, but not dealt with at length since their management usually becomes the prerogative of the specialist neurological unit.

This book is designed to be relatively easy armchair reading for the general practitioner, senior medical student or others who may be interested in the mechanism of headache or concerned with the practical management of headache problems. The neurologist may find something of interest in the chapters on tension headache and migraine. References are listed for those who wish to read in greater depth.

The present concept of headache mechanisms depends to a great extent on the work of the late Harold G. Wolff and his colleagues, which is described in Wolff's monograph *Headache and other Head Pain*. The reader is referred to this work for aspects of headache which are passed over lightly here. The subject may not have all the excitement of a detective story but the talents of the great detectives of fiction would not be lost in trying to unravel some of the complexities of headache.

J. W. L.

Preface to the Second Edition

In the three years since the appearance of the first edition sufficient research work has been done on vascular headache to warrant considerable revision of the text. The greatest changes have taken place in the understanding of migraine, particularly the nature of hormonal influences on premenstrual migraine and the mechanism of action of new pharmaceutical agents for the control of migraine. Cluster headache (migrainous neuralgia) has now been culled from the migrainous fold and granted the dignity of a chapter to itself. Minor alterations have been made throughout the book to bring each section into line with current thought. Seventy references have been added, but 57 have been deleted to preserve the quality of ease of reading. References have been removed, not because they are necessarily outdated but because, for the most part, they were essential for the documentation of facts which are now generally accepted. The author hopes that the new text has gained in authority, while remaining comfortable to hold lightly in one hand.

Sydney, N.S.W.   James W. Lance

Acknowledgements

Many of the studies in migraine which are described in this book were undertaken by Donald A. Curran, MD, Michael Anthony, MD, Brian W. Somerville, MD, Paul J. Spira, MD, and George Lord, MD, during the tenure of a research fellowship in neurology provided by Sandoz (Australia) Ltd., in the author's department. The research programme owes much to the advice and help of Herta Hinterberger, PhD, DSc, Senior Research Officer, Division of Clinical Chemistry, The Prince Henry Hospital, Sydney, and is being continued by Dr Anthony, Dr E. J. Mylecharane and Mr J. W. Duckworth. I am grateful to my neurosurgical colleagues for years of friendly collaboration in managing headache and other problems.

I wish to thank my secretary, Mrs R. M. Kendall, for her willing and efficient assistance, which always makes my tasks a lot lighter. My thanks are also due to Miss B. Pate, Librarian, for obtaining all references.

The anatomical diagrams were made by Mrs F. Rubiu and Mr J. Elliott Watson. All photographs and figures were prepared by the Department of Medical Illustration, University of New South Wales.

I am grateful to the editors of the following publications for permission to reproduce figures from some of my earlier papers: *Medical Journal of Australia; Journal of Neurology, Neurosurgery and Psychiatry; Archives of Neurology; Research and Clinical Studies in Headache* (Karger of Basel and New York); *Headache* and the *Journal of Neurological Sciences*. Figures are reproduced from Dr Somerville's papers on hormonal changes in migraine by courtesy of the editors of *Neurology*.

The research programme has been supported throughout by the National Health and Medical Research Council of Australia.

One

Causes of Headache

A CONSIDERATION OF PAIN PATHWAYS AND GENERAL MECHANISMS OF HEADACHE

The question 'why does the head ache?' is not as naïve as it appears at first. The brain, the ependymal lining of the ventricles and choroid plexuses within the brain and much of the dura and pia-arachnoid which cover the convexity of the brain are insensitive to pain. The floor of the anterior and posterior fossa gives rise to pain on stimulation but the middle cranial fossa is sensitive only in the vicinity of the middle meningeal artery. Direct pressure on cranial nerves which carry pain fibres will of course give rise to pain, but this is an uncommon event. The most important structures which register intracranial pain are the vessels, particularly the proximal part of the cerebral and dural arteries, and the large veins and venous sinuses (Ray and Wolff, 1940). A fever or 'hangover' gives rise to a throbbing headache because the cerebral arteries are dilated. An expanding lesion in one hemisphere (for example haematoma, abscess or tumour) produces headache by displacing vessels, often pushing the anterior cerebral arteries across the midline. Rapid enlargement of the ventricles, caused by internal hydrocephalus from obstruction of the cerebrospinal fluid (CSF) pathways, thrusts vessels outwards symmetrically. Oedema of the cerebral hemispheres displaces centrally placed vessels inwards as well, since the ventricles become smaller because of pressure from the swollen brain. When the pressure of CSF, which helps maintain the brain in its normal position, is lowered by lumbar puncture, the brain may pull on its supporting structures and cause headache by traction on the intracranial vessels. Because of their vascular origin, all forms of intracranial headache tend to throb with the pulse, more especially on exertion, and

1

are made worse by any sudden jolt or jar, or with coughing, sneezing or straining.

Pain from the dura

Pain from the upper surface of the tentorium and the anterior and middle cranial fossae is transmitted by the trigeminal nerve. A recurrent branch of the trigeminal nerve arises from the first (ophthalmic) division near its origin and supplies the superior surface of the tentorium and the falx, so that pain from vessels in these areas of dura is readily referred to the eye and forehead of the same side. Afferent fibres from the middle meningeal artery are of trigeminal origin, mainly from the second and third divisions (McNaughton, 1937). The tentorium is the watershed for dural innervation since its inferior surface and the whole of the posterior fossa is supplied chiefly by the upper three cervical nerve roots and so refers pain to the back of the head and upper part of the neck. The ninth and tenth cranial nerves supply part of the posteria fossa and thus pain may sometimes be referred to the ear or throat. The result of the innervation of the dura and its vessels, in brief, is that pain from supratentorial structures is referred to the anterior two-thirds of the head by the trigeminal nerve and pain from infratentorial structures is referred to the back of the head and neck by the upper cervical nerve roots (*Figures 1.1 and 1.2*).

Pain from cerebral arteries

Apart from the vessels of the dura, the larger proximal parts of the intracerebral arteries are sensitive to stimulation and refer pain to the eye, forehead or temple of the same side (Fay, 1937). During carotid angiography under local anaesthesia, the injection of contrast medium into the internal carotid artery is signalled by pain felt deeply behind the eye. The pain of intracranial vascular headache induced by histamine depends upon the integrity of the trigeminal nerve. Blood pressure responses elicited in the monkey by stimulating the vicinity of cortical arteries are abolished by section of the trigeminal nerve (Wall and Pribram, 1950). It therefore seems logical that pain from the intracranial arteries is mediated in some way by the trigeminal nerve but the pathway concerned remains an anatomical puzzle.

The nerve plexus which surrounds the internal and external carotid systems in man is almost entirely of sympathetic origin from the eighth cervical and the first, second and third thoracic segments of the spinal cord via the superior cervical ganglion. There is a small parasympathetic contribution from the facial nerve through the greater superficial petrosal nerve (Chorobski and Penfield, 1932). Both internal and external carotid nerve plexuses contain some myelinated fibres of larger calibre than those of sympathetic origin, which are thought to be afferent fibres of the vagus nerve and upper thoracic spinal nerves (Kuntz, 1934; Kuntz, Hoffman and Napolitano, 1957). In the region

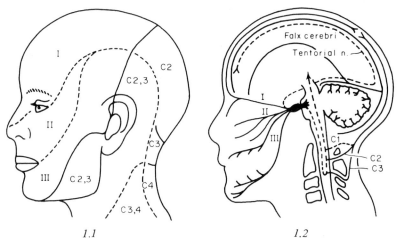

1.1   *1.2*

Figure 1.1. Cutaneous distribution of the trigeminal nerve to the face and anterior two-thirds of the scalp, showing the watershed with the cervical nerves above the ear line (after Cunningham)

Figure 1.2. Schematic representation of the three divisions of the trigeminal nerve, the Gasserian ganglion and the upper cervical nerve roots. Attention is drawn to three interrupted lines. One line indicates the path taken by the spinal tract and nucleus of the trigeminal nerve as it descends into the upper cervical segments of the cord. Afferent fibres from the first, second and third cervical nerve roots and the trigeminal pathway converge upon some cells in the posterior horns of the spinal cord, thus permitting referral of pain from neck to head and vice versa. The crossed second-order neurones pass upwards to the thalamus. Another interrupted line indicates the course of the tentorial nerve. The first cervical nerve root is represented by an interrupted line because it is inconstant

of the carotid sinus, the internal carotid plexus receives twigs from the third, fourth and sixth cranial nerves, but there is no evidence of any constant communication with the fifth (trigeminal) nerve to account for the distribution of pain from the internal carotid artery and its branches to the anterior part of the head (Fang, 1961). There is clinical evidence that some pain fibres from these vessels may take a long route home by descending in the perivascular plexus and then accompanying sympathetic nerve fibres to the upper thoracic and lower cervical spinal cord. Fay (1937) described headache persisting in spite of division of the trigeminal, glossopharyngeal and vagal nerves as well as the upper three cervical nerve roots. The headache which survived such extensive surgical measures finally disappeared when spinal anaesthesia was induced and extended upwards until it involved the eighth cervical segment with the onset of numbness on the ulnar aspects of the hands. This supports the anatomical evidence of afferent fibres descending in the carotid plexus to enter the spinal cord, but the part which these play in the appreciation of vascular headache has not been established.

The vertebral arterial plexus is less constant than that of the carotid system. Fang (1961) demonstrated that innervation was solely uni-lateral in over two-thirds of human subjects. Small contributions to the vertebrobasilar plexus are made from the third, fifth, seventh, ninth, eleventh and twelfth cranial nerves.

Pain from extracranial arteries

The scalp arteries comprise the supra-orbital, frontal, superficial temporal, postauricular and occipital arteries, all of which receive filaments from adjacent cutaneous nerves. Ray and Wolff (1940) showed that these arteries were sensitive to stimulation and stretching and were able to produce a throbbing headache by rhythmically distending and collapsing the superficial temporal artery. If several portions of the artery were distended together, the subject became nauseated. When the nerves around the scalp arteries were blocked with a local anaesthetic agent, the whole vessel did not become numb, indicating that there were multiple sources of nerve supply to the artery throughout its length. Pain is experienced in the immediate neighbour-hood of an artery which is inflamed or distended. Pain from the supra-orbital, frontal and superficial temporal arteries is mediated by the trigeminal nerve, and from the postauricular and occipital arteries by the upper cervical nerve roots.

Pain from the skull, sinuses, eyes, teeth and neck

The cranial bones are insensitive, but stretch of the periosteum evokes pain locally. Pain from the eye, nasal sinuses and teeth is felt locally at first, then may be referred to the appropriate division of the trigeminal nerve, with some overflow to adjacent divisions if the pain is severe.

Diffuse headache from contraction of head and neck muscles may follow later if local pain is sustained. The whole pattern then assumes the character of tension headache and muscular overaction can be demonstrated by electromyography (Wolff, 1963).

Degenerative changes in the upper cervical spine may cause compression of the first, second and third cervical nerve roots with referral of pain to the back of the head. Pain from a cervical disc lesion may rarely be referred to one eye and one half of the head, probably because some afferent fibres from the first and second cervical nerve roots converge upon cells in the posterior horn of the spinal cord, which can also be excited by trigeminal afferent fibres (Kerr, 1961a), thus conveying to the patient the impression of head pain through this shared pathway. Stimulation of the first, but not the second, cervical posterior root consistently gives rise to frontal and orbital pain in man (Kerr, 1961b). Wolff mentions that the second and third nerve roots may refer pain to the vertex. There is no known way for lesions of the lower cervical spine to cause pain in the head other than by producing overaction of the head and neck muscles, presumably in a subconscious or reflex attempt to prevent neck movement.

Muscle-contraction or 'tension' headache can be relieved by the infiltration of local anaesthetic into the affected muscle and is mediated by the trigeminal nerve or the upper cervical nerve roots.

Central pathways for head pain

Pain fibres from all three divisions of the trigeminal nerve descend in the spinal tract of the trigeminal nerve to the second cervical segment in a laminated fashion, the ophthalmic fibres lying ventrolaterally and the mandibular fibres lying dorsomedially (Selby, 1975). They are joined in their path by pain fibres from the facial nerve (nervus intermedius), glossopharyngeal and vagus nerves. Recent work has shown that the upper segments of the spinal cord form an important centre for the relay of head pain since the spinal tract and nucleus of the trigeminal nerve plunge down to the region of entry of the upper cervical roots which supply the occipital region and upper neck. Sensory fibres from the upper three cervical dorsal roots ramify throughout this centre and make some synaptic contact with trigeminal neurones in the spinal nucleus, which permits referral of pain from the upper neck to the head and vice versa (*see Figure 1.2*).

There is much greater overlap between the trigeminal and cervical distribution than was previously realized. Denny-Brown and Yanagisawa (1973) sectioned the sensory root of one trigeminal nerve in a monkey and found the expected sensory loss over the anterior two-thirds of the face and scalp. When the animal was given a subconvulsive dose of strychnine, the area of anaesthesia receded until the only unresponsive region was around the eye, cheek and upper lip, apparently the only area innervated exclusively by the fifth cranial nerve. Conversely, section of the second, third and fourth cervical dorsal roots produced a sensory loss over the occipital region and upper neck, which shrank to a thin band around the neck after strychnine. When trigeminal and cervical inflow were both destroyed, there was still an area of innervation by the vagus and facial nerves around the ear which spread in a wedge shape to supply the posterior half of the scalp under the influence of strychnine. It has not been appreciated that the vagus nerve, through its communication with auriculotemporal and posterior temporal branches, supplies the ear and a large part of the scalp. Normal input from two sources is presumably required to stimulate cells of the spinal nucleus but one source is sufficient under the influence of strychnine. It remains to be seen whether this can be applied to the patient with headache.

The rostral part of the spinal tract and nucleus of the trigeminal nerve (nucleus oralis) is concerned with pain impulses from a limited area around the eye, nose and lips because section of the tract at the pontomedullary junction spares this area. Fibres from all three divisions descend to the upper spinal cord. After synapsing, the second-order neurones cross the midline and ascend through the brainstem as the quintothalamic tract to the posteroventromedial nucleus of the thalamus.

Endorphins

A new approach to the study of pain has followed the discovery that opiates bind selectively to the membranes of cells in various parts of the nervous system. Naturally occurring substances which use the same receptor sites and which may influence transmission in central pain pathways have now been identified and have been called endorphins (endogenous morphine-like substances). Endorphins are polypeptides with the same aminoacid sequence as beta-lipotropin, a component of pituitary extracts. Active fragments of endorphins are known as enkephalins. Short-chain polypeptides are distributed widely throughout the central nervous system, including the median raphe of the brainstem and the dorsal horn of spinal cord. If these substances prove to be inhibitory transmitters responsible for the regulation of pain pathways, any deficiency in them might account for some syndromes of spontaneous pain. Future developments in this field will have important applications to the problem of headache.

Control of the cranial blood vessels

Because pain from both extra-and intracranial arteries plays such an important part in headache, it is important to understand the way in which the calibre of these vessels is controlled. Under normal conditions, cerebral blood flow (CBF) remains constant irrespective of a wide variation in perfusion pressure. If the blood pressure increases while intracranial pressure is unaltered, the arteries constrict to maintain normal flow. Conversely, they dilate when blood pressure drops. This response, known as autogenic regulation, is a reaction of the smooth muscle cells of the arteriolar wall independent of autonomic innervation. Autoregulation is abolished in cerebral ischaemia (including the ischaemia induced by migraine) and also by the infusion of prostaglandin E_1, a vasodilator substance which can provoke a migraine attack in normal subjects. Increase in arterial pCO_2 (hypercapnia) exerts a profound dilator influence on cerebral vessels while hypocapnia causes vasoconstriction, probably mediated by the bicarbonate concentration in the cerebrospinal fluid surrounding arterioles (Lassen, 1974). The vasoconstrictor effect of hypocapnia depends upon an intact sympathetic nerve supply (Corbett, Eidelman and Debarge, 1972).

Neural control

The pial arteries are innervated by sympathetic fibres originating in the superior cervical ganglion. Small arterial branches in the brain parenchyma of the rat have a separate noradrenergic innervation which does not travel in a perivascular plexus but passes directly from the brainstem, mainly from the locus coeruleus (Hartman, Zide and Udenfriend, 1972). This brings up the possibility of the cortical microcirculation being regulated independently of the parent arteries. Parasympathetic fibres reach the pial arteries from the greater superficial petrosal branch of the facial nerve. Most studies report a modest (5 – 10 per cent) decrease or increase in cerebral blood flow on maximal stimulation of sympathetic or parasympathetic fibres respectively (Lassen, 1974). In one study, blood flow in the internal carotid artery of the monkey was shown to diminish by as much as 30 per cent with sympathetic stimulation (Meyer, Yoshida and Sakamoto, 1967). However, section of the cervical sympathetic does not increase cerebral blood flow or oxygen availability in cat or monkey, suggesting that the sympathetic nervous system is not responsible for maintaining vasomotor tone. This is consistent with observations in man that stellate ganglion blockade, unilateral or bilateral, does not augment cerebral blood flow.

The effect of sympathetic stimulation is greater on extracranial vessels, causing a decrease in oxygen availability in the temporalis muscle in cat and monkey, and reducing blood flow in the monkey external carotid by about 68 per cent (Meyer, Yoshida and Sakamoto, 1967). It is doubtful whether this action has any physiological significance since the forehead and scalp are not susceptible to the sort of vasoconstrictor reflexes that are seen in the hands and feet. Startle, immersion of the hand in iced water, or taking a deep breath do not affect pulsation in forehead skin. The vascular reactions of the forehead are like those of a sympathectomized digit in that constriction is gradual as skin temperature falls, probably because of the direct effect of cold on the vessels (Hertzman and Roth, 1942). Heat loss from the forehead remains constant during body cooling while heat loss from the fingers decreases by a factor of six (Froese and Burton, 1957). Unilateral cervicodorsal ganglionectomy results in a consistent rise in skin temperature in the limbs, but not in the face or scalp. Blocking the cervical sympathetic in three subjects, of whom the author was one, did not increase the amplitude of pulsation of the superficial temporal artery. There is little increase in heat flow after blockade of scalp nerves (Fox, Goldsmith and Kidd, 1962).

It is therefore evident that the sympathetic nervous system plays little part in maintaining tonic constriction of scalp vessels. On the other hand, it is known to be important in vasodilator reflexes. Capillary dilator fibres pass from the anterior thoracolumbar nerve roots and sympathetic ganglia and are distributed to vessels of the scalp and forehead. There is evidence that some vasodilator fibres pass out in the trigeminal nerve (Oka, 1950). Blushing is abolished by sympathectomy, and flushing of the scalp and forehead no longer occurs in response to overheating of the body after sympathectomy or blockade of the cutaneous nerve supply to those areas (Fox, Goldsmith and Kidd, 1962).

Humoral control

Humoral control of the cranial vessels has been studied extensively in recent years in a variety of animals. In our own observations on the monkey (Spira, Mylecharane and Lance, 1976), serotonin, noradrenaline, adrenaline and prostaglandin $F_{2\alpha}$ produced vasoconstriction in both internal and external carotid arteries, the effects being much more conspicuous in the external carotid circulation. Bradykinin and histamine dilated both circulations. Acetyl choline had little effect on the internal carotid artery but dilated the external carotid circulation. Prostaglandin E_1 produced marked external carotid dilatation while flow in the internal carotid artery was actually reduced, possibly as a 'steal' phenomenon because of reduction of pressure in the common carotid artery reducing perfusion pressure. Other authors have reported conflicting results on the effect of prostaglandin E_1 on the intracranial circulation.

Serotonin constricts the external carotid vascular bed in dog and man as well as in the monkey (Spira, Mylecharane and Lance, 1976) but acts as a vasodilator in the baboon (Grimson et al., 1969). Since there is no obvious difference in the experimental techniques employed, it must be assumed that this is a species variation. Carroll, Ebeling and Glover (1974) found that serotonin was a more potent constrictor of the human temporal artery than was noradrenaline. It is thought that serotonin may be important in maintaining tonic vasoconstriction of the extracranial vessels in normal man but this is by no means certain.

Alpha and beta adrenergic receptors are present in the middle cerebral artery of the cat (Edvinsson and Owman, 1974), responsible for constriction and dilatation respectively, but we have not been able to demonstrate beta effects in the monkey circulation. Recent evidence suggests that vasodilatation in response to β-adrenergic or chemical stimuli is associated with an increase in intracellular $3'$, $5'$- adenosine monophosphate (cyclic AMP) (Flamm et al., 1975). A neurotransmitter or drug activates the enzyme adenylate cyclase which acts on adenosine triphosphate (ATP) in the presence of Mg^{++} to form cyclic AMP. Cyclic AMP appears to act by reducing available Ca^{++} which is necessary for vasoconstriction. Cyclic AMP remains active until it is hydrolyzed by cAMP-phospho-diesterase (PDE) to form $5'$-AMP.

The dilatation produced by histamine can be mediated through histamine-1 receptors, which are responsible for the drop in blood pressure when histamine is infused and are blocked by conventional antihistaminic drugs. It may also be mediated by histamine-2 receptors, one variety of which is responsible for the stimulation of secretion of gastric acid by histamine, that is blocked by metiamide and cimetidine but not by the usual antihistamines. Our studies (Duckworth et al., 1976) in the monkey have shown that the intracranial circulation contains both H_1 and H_2 receptors but that the extracranial arteries have mainly H_2 receptors. This is also true for the dog (Saxena,

1975) as well as for human temporal artery and has obvious implications for therapy in headache.

Recent work by Edvinsson and Hardebo (1976) has indicated that there may be specific serotonin receptors in the extracranial circulation of cat and man responsible for vasoconstriction which are inhibited competitively by methysergide. When the vessels were constricted tonically by the addition of $PGE_{2\alpha}$, serotonin acted as a vasodilator in both intracranial and extracranial arteries, the effect being greater intracranially. This dilation was blocked by propranolol and not methysergide, showing that it depended upon beta-adrenergic receptors. These contrasting effects of serotonin, depending upon the pre-existing state of constriction of the vessel and the type of receptor present, may account for the fact that the baboon extracranial circulation responds differently to serotonin from that of dog, monkey and man. The place of vasoactive substances in the normal control of the circulation is not yet established but there is strong evidence to implicate them in the pathogenesis of vascular headache which will be presented in later chapters.

SUMMARY

The scalp vessels, cranial periosteum and dura are innervated chiefly by the trigeminal nerve over the anterior two-thirds of the head, and by the upper three cervical nerve roots over the posterior third. Displacement or dilatation of intracranial vessels and distension of extracranial arteries are common causes of headache. It is not certain which pain pathways serve the sensitive basal portion of the intracranial arteries, although the areas to which pain is referred are in the trigeminal distribution. There is evidence that some pain fibres descend with the periarterial nerve plexuses in the neck to reach the lower cervical and upper thoracic spinal cord, but the role of these fibres in headache is uncertain.

Overlap between the projection of afferent fibres in the upper cervical nerve roots and those of the trigeminal nerve offer an explanation for the referral of pain to the head in disorders of the upper cervical spine. Sensory connections of the vagus and facial nerves ramify over the posterior half of the scalp in the monkey but whether these nerves play any part in headache in man is unknown. Neural and humoral control of blood vessels must be considered in relation to the vascular changes in headache.

Neural control of cranial and extracranial blood vessels is mediated almost entirely by the sympathetic nervous system. There is no evidence of tonic vasoconstrictor action on these vessels except in the ear, which appears to have a different control mechanism from the scalp and forehead and cerebral vessels. Vasoconstriction may be induced experimentally by stimulation of the cervical sympathetic trunk, more so in extracranial than intracranial vessels, but it is doubtful whether this has physiological significance since vasoconstrictor reflexes are virtually absent from forehead and scalp. In contrast, vasodilator reflexes are active in these areas and depend upon sympathetic fibres travelling with cutaneous nerves. Small arterial branches in the rat brain have a direct noradrenergic innervation from the brainstem, which means that the cortical microcirculation may be regulated independently of the parent arteries.

The cranial vessels are extremely sensitive to humoral agents. In monkey and man, serotonin, noradrenaline, adrenaline and prostaglandin $F_{2\alpha}$ are vasoconstrictors, particularly of the external carotid circulation. Bradykinin, histamine and prostaglandin E_1 dilate both circulations. Vasodilatation is associated with an increase in intracellular cyclic AMP. The dilatation induced by histamine depends upon both H_1 and H_2 receptors in the intracranial circulation but mainly H_2 receptors in the extracranial arteries. These findings have obvious implications in the cause and treatment of vascular headaches.

REFERENCES

Carroll, P.R., Ebeling, P.W. and Glover, W.E. (1974). The responses of the human temporal and rabbit ear artery to 5-hydroxytryptamine and some of its antagonists. *Aust. J. exp. Biol. med. Sci.* **52**, 813

Chorobski, J. and Penfield, W. (1932). Cerebral vasodilator nerves and their pathway from the medulla oblongata. *Archs Neurol. Psychiat., Chicago* **28**, 1257

Corbett, J.L., Eidelman, B.H. and Debarge, O. (1972). Modification of cerebral vasoconstriction with hyperventilation in normal man with thymoxamine. *Lancet* **2**, 461

Denny-Brown, D. and Yanagisawa, N. (1973). The function of the descending root of the fifth nerve. *Brain* **96**, 783

Duckworth, J.W., Lance, J.W., Lord, G.D.A. and Mylecharane, E.J. (1976). Histamine receptors in the cranial circulation of the monkey. *Br. J. Pharmac.* **58**, 444p.

Edvinsson, L. and Hardebo, J.E. (1976). Characterization of serotonin receptors in intracranial and extracranial vessels. Abstr. Int. Symp. Sept 16–17. London: Migraine Trust, 12

Edvinsson, L. and Owman, C. (1974). Pharmacological characterization of adrenergic alpha and beta receptors mediating the vasomotor responses of cerebral arteries in vitro. *Circulation Res.* **35**, 835

Fang, H.C.H. (1961). Cerebral arterial innervations in man. *Archs Neurol.* **4**, 651

Fay, T. (1937). Mechanism of headache. *Archs Neurol. Psychiat., Chicago* **37**, 471

Flamm, E.S., Kim, J., Lin, J. and Ransohoff, J. (1975). Phosphodiesterase inhibitors and cerebral vasospasm. *Archs. Neurol.* **32**, 569

Fox, R.H., Goldsmith, R. and Kidd, D.J. (1962). Cutaneous vasomotor control in the human head, neck and upper chest. *J. Physiol.* **161**, 298

Froese, G. and Burton, A.C. (1957). Heat losses from the human head. *J. appl. Physiol.* **10**, 235

Grimson, B.S., Robinson, S.C., Danford, E.T., Tindall, G.T. and Greenfield, J.C. Jr (1969) Effect of serotonin on internal and external carotid artery blood flow in the baboon. *Am. J. Physiol.* **216**, 50

Hartman, B.K., Zide, D. and Udenfriend, S. (1972). The use of dopamine β-hydroxylase as a marker for the central noradrenergic nervous system in rat brain. *Proc. natn. Acad. Sci. U.S.A.* **69**, 2722

Hertzman, A.B. and Roth, L.W. (1942). The absence of vasoconstrictor reflexes in the forehead circulation. Effects of cold. *Am. J. Physiol.* **136**, 692

Kerr, F.W.L. (1961a). Trigeminal and cervical volleys. *Archs Neurol.* **5**, 171

Kerr, F.W.L. (1961b). A mechanism to account for frontal headache in cases of posterior fossa tumours. *J. Neurosurg.* **18**, 605

Kuntz, A. (1934). Nerve fibres of spinal and vagus origin associated with the cephalic sympathetic nerves. *Ann. Otol. Rhinol. Lar.* **43**, 50

Kuntz, A., Hoffman, H. H. and Napolitano, L.M. (1957). Cephalic sympathetic nerves. *Archs surg.* **75**, 108

Lassen, N.A. (1974). Control of cerebral circulation in health and disease. *Circulation Res.* **34**, 749

McNaughton, F.L. (1937). The innervation of the intracranial blood vessels and dural sinuses. *Proc. Ass. Res. nerv. ment. Dis.* **18**, 178

Meyer, J.S., Yoshida, K. and Sakamoto, K. (1967). Autonomic control of cerebral blood flow measured by electromagnetic flowmeters. *Neurology, Minneap.* **17**, 638

Oka, M. (1950). Experimental study on the vasodilator innervation of the face. *Med. J. Osaka Univ.* **2**, 109

Ray, B.S. and Wolff, H.G. (1940). Experimental studies on headache. Pain sensitive structures of the head and their significance in headache. *Archs Surg.* **41**, 813

Saxena, P.R. (1975). Two types of histamine receptors in a vascular bed of relevance to migrainous headache. In *Vasoactive Substances Relevant to Migraine* (Ed. S. Diamond, D.J. Dalessio, J. R. Graham and J. L. Medina. p. 34. Springfield Ill.: Thomas

Selby, G. (1975). Diseases of the fifth cranial nerve. In *Peripheral Neuropathy* p.533. Philadelphia: Saunders

Spira, P.J., Mylecharane, E.J. and Lance, J.W. (1976). The effects of humoral agents and antimigraine drugs on the cranial circulation of the monkey. *Res. clin. Stud. Headache (Basel/Karger)*, **4**, 37

Wall, P.D. and Pribram, K.H. (1950). Trigeminal neurotomy and blood pressure responses from stimulation of lateral cerebral cortex of *Macaca mulata*. *J. Neurophysiol.* **13**, 409

Wolff, H.G. (1963). *Headache and Other Head Pain*. New York: Oxford University Press

Two
Classification of Headache and Facial Pain

The consideration of pain pathways and mechanisms involved in the perception of headache leads naturally to thoughts on the classification of headache. Headache may be divided into groups on the grounds of site, rapidity of onset, association with neurological signs and many other clinical criteria. Such categories help in differential diagnosis and will be used for this purpose later on. The most useful classification of the many varieties of headache to precede individual clinical description is one which is based as far as possible on knowledge of pain mechanisms.

The classification presented here, which is modified from the recommendations of the Ad Hoc Committee on Classification of Headache, (Friedman *et al.*, 1962) starts with those forms of headache and facial pain which have a clearly recognizable organic cause. Once these have been eliminated there are entities such as classical migraine and cluster headache with a distinctive clinical syndrome and pathophysiology which can be placed readily in separate categories. When one comes to common migraine, tension-vascular headache, tension headache and 'ordinary headaches', there is often difficulty in defining the line of demarcation precisely, particularly as this process depends almost entirely on the history given by the patient. Attempts at history-taking and symptom analysis by computer have run into the same difficulties experienced by the clinician (Ziegler, Hassanein and Hassanein, 1972). The listing of categories here is not meant to imply that there is not some overlap between the various forms of functional headache or some common factor underlying them.

13

Local cranial disorders

1. Expanding lesions within the cranial bones stretching the periosteum.
2. Inflammation of the cranium or scalp.
3. Temporal arteritis.
4. Carotidynia.

Pain from the cranial nerves

1. Excessive stimulation of trigeminal or glossopharyngeal nerves (e.g. ice-cream headache).
2. Compression or inflammation of cranial nerves.
   Tumour, aneurysm.
   Tolosa-Hunt syndrome.
   Raeder's paratrigeminal neuralgia.
   Gradenigo's syndrome.
   Post-herpetic neuralgia.
   Central lesions, multiple sclerosis.
3. Trigeminal or glossopharyngeal neuralgia.
4. Atypical facial pain of unknown aetiology.

Referred pain

1. Eyes: eye strain, retrobulbar neuritis, glaucoma.
2. Ear, nose and throat: sinusitis, nasopharyngeal carcinoma.
3. Teeth: apical root abscess, temporomandibular joint dysfunction (Costen's syndrome).
4. Neck: cervical spondylosis, rheumatoid arthritis

Intracranial sources of headache

1. Vasodilatation, the cause of which may be:
   (a) toxic, for example systemic infections, 'hangover', carbon monoxide poisoning, caffeine withdrawal, foreign protein reactions, indomethacin medication.
   (b) metabolic, for example hypoxia, hypoglycaemia, hypercapnia.
   (c) vasodilator agents such as histamine, nitrites or monosodium glutamate.

(d) postconcussional.

(e) postconvulsive.

(f) acute pressor reactions, such as the headache produced by phaeochromocytoma, tyramine ingestion by a patient taking mono-amine oxidase inhibitors; sexual excitement; or

(g) essential hypertension.

2. Meningeal irritation, as in subarachnoid haemorrhage, meningitis, encephalitis, postpneumo-encephalographic or postmyelographic reactions.

3. Traction on, or displacement of, intracranial vessels.
This may be due to:

(a) space-occupying lesions, such as tumour, haematoma or abscess.

(b) increased intracranial pressure, for example blockage of CSF pathways (hydrocephalus), superior sagittal or lateral sinus thrombosis (otitic hydrocephalus), raised venous pressure (emphysema, mediastinal obstruction) cerebral oedema from other causes (post-craniotomy, acute nephritis, malignant hypertension, 'benign intracranial hypertension', hypocalcaemia, adrenal corticosteroids, Addison's disease); or

(c) reduced intracranial pressure, as in post-lumbar puncture headache.

4. Exertional and cough headache of benign aetiology.

Episodic vascular headaches

1. Vascular headache of migraine type, which may be common migraine, classical migraine, basilar artery migraine, retinal migraine, hemiplegic migraine, ophthalmoplegic migraine, facial migraine ('lower half headache'), migraine equivalents.

2. Cluster headache (migrainous neuralgia).

3. Acute cerebral vascular insufficiency.

Muscle-contraction headache

1. Secondary to other factors, as in eyestrain, imbalance of bite, cervical spondylosis.

2. Primary muscle overaction (tension headache).

3. Combination with vascular headache (tension-vascular headache).

Post-traumatic headaches

These comprise an important aetiological category but their mechanism embraces vascular, neural and psychological factors which could lead to their classification under a number of the above headings.

Psychogenic headache

Depressive, delusional, conversion or hypochondriacal states.

REFERENCES

Friedman, A.P., Finley, K.M., Graham, J.R., Kunkle, E.C., Ostfeld, A.M. and Wolff, H.G. (1962). Classification of headache. The Ad Hoc Committee on the Classification of Headache, *Archs Neurol.* **6**, 173

Ziegler, D.K., Hassanein, R. and Hassanein, K. (1972). Headache syndromes suggested by a factor analysis of symptom variables in a headache-prone population. *J. chron. Dis.* **25**, 353

Three

Recording the History

The diagnostic battle is often lost or won in the first skirmish. If a patient complaining of headache or facial pain is first seen in a busy office or general clinic, with a background noise of coughing and shuffling feet from the waiting room, it is probably better to make an appointment for another time when the problem can be discussed in detail. If sufficient time is given to the initial interview, the majority of patients can be assessed adequately without recourse to special investigations. A careful systematic history will enable one to make a firm diagnosis of some disorders such as cluster headache and tic douloureux and to make a provisional diagnosis in most patients with tension headache, migraine, sinusitis, ocular disturbance or cervical spondylosis. The evolution of the headache may raise suspicions of more serious conditions such as subdural haematoma, cerebral tumour or temporal arteritis. The history is much more important than physical examination, which is often completely normal in patients with headache.

The most convenient form for the history is the same as that used to gather information about pain elsewhere in the body. When the essential points are always written down in the same order under the same headings, a pattern of headache emerges in the shortest possible time which is often sufficient to make the diagnosis. The writing of a long narrative in the rambling or disconnected sequence dictated by a loquacious patient is an interesting literary exercise for those with time on their hands. It has the disadvantage that the diagnostic pattern of the story may be obscured and that if the patient should be subject to more than one kind of headache, the strands of each may become hopelessly interwoven in the verbal loom. History-taking by computer runs into the same problems (Stead *et al.*, 1972) but may yet prove to be a time-saving preliminary step in large clinics.

17

The following excerpt from the casebook of a well-known physician makes some important points but is not complete enough to permit of diagnosis with certainty:

> Most of the time he seemed to see something shining before him like a light, usually in part of the right eye; at the end of a moment, a violent pain supervened in the right temple, then in all the head and neck, where the head is attached to the spine ... vomiting, when it became possible, was able to divert the pain and render it more moderate.

A more elaborate description of a headache syndrome, written in discursive style, still omits information which we would like to have:

> In certain cases, the parts on the right side, or those on the left solely, so far that a separate temple, or ear, or one eyebrow, or one eye, or the nose which divides the face into two equal parts; and the pain does not pass this limit, but remains in the half of the head. This is called Heterocrania, an illness by no means mild, even though it intermits and although it appears to be slight. For if at any time it set in acutely, it occasions unseemly and dreadful symptoms; spasm and distortion of the countenance takes place; the eyes either fixed intently like horns, or they are rolled inwardly to this side or to that; vertigo, deep-seated pain of the eyes as far as the meninges; irre-strainable sweat; sudden pain of the tendons, as of one striking with a club; nausea; vomiting of bilious matters; collapse of the patient ... there is much torpor, heaviness of the head, anxiety, and ennui. For they flee the light; the darkness soothes their disease: nor can they bear readily to look upon or hear anything agreeable; their sense of smell is vitiated, neither does anything agreeable to smell delight them; and they have also an aversion to fetid things: The patients, moreover, are weary of life, and wish to die.

The first description was written by Hippocrates (Critchley, 1967) about 400 B.C. and the second by Aretaeus of Cappadocia (Adams, 1841) about A.D. 150. The vividness of imagery leaves little doubt that both were depicting migraine, although other disorders may have crept in to Aretaeus' account. Since the average medical man is not writing his case histories for posterity, greater economy of style may be granted to him and a systematic record will give a clearer, if less elegant, picture of the patient's illness. It is often of assistance to quote directly any phrase of the patient's which appears well-chosen and likely to throw light on the illness.

There would still be notable gaps in the record of these headaches of antiquity if the above quotations were combined and transcribed in summary, as follows;

Length of illness:	unstated
Frequency of headache:	unstated
Duration of headache:	unstated
Site of headache:	half head, right or left, maximal in temple, eye or frontal region, radiating to ear, nostril and neck.
Quality of headache:	'violent' (constant or pulsating?)
Time of onset:	unstated
Mode of onset:	light shining in part of right eye (in right half of visual field?) lasting a moment
Associated features:	nausea, vomiting, photophobia, disturbed sense of smell, sweating, vertigo, aching limbs, anxiety, depression, and drowsiness. Collapse (syncopal attack? epileptic in view of eyes rolling?)
Precipitating factors:	unstated. (We could here insert 'drinking wine . . . or heat of a fire, or the sun', by borrowing from the Roman physician Cornelius Celsus, a friend of the Emperor Tiberius (Critchley, 1967).
Relieving factors:	darkness, vomiting. Specific therapy (namely, bleeding and the use of hellebore) is mentioned elsewhere by Hippocrates (Critchley, 1967).

This analysis gives a vivid picture of migraine (with some atypical features) but is not helpful in establishing the temporal pattern of attacks which is so important in diagnosis, and in the timing of treatment to prevent attacks. The temporal pattern also serves as a baseline on which to assess the results of therapy. If the patient is subject to bouts of headache lasting for several weeks followed by freedom from headache for months, one obviously has to be careful about interpreting a remission as the result of treatment. Lack of knowledge of the natural history of cluster headache was responsible for cures being attributed to histamine desensitization, while in fact the natural periodicity of the disorder remained unaltered by treatment. Any serious assessment of results must be controlled by the use of a placebo or an alternative treatment without the knowledge of either patient or physician of which treatment they are being given until after their response is documented. This sort of procedure is unnecessary in normal clinical practice but a healthy and critical scepticism must be maintained as any disorder fluctuates in intensity and remission may easily be abetted by the enthusiastic adoption of a new method of treatment.

To assist diagnosis of headache and help plan treatment it is thus worthwhile to have standard headings, such as those which have just been applied impiously to Hippocrates and Aretaeus.

At the top of the history sheet, the presenting symptom may be written as:

Headaches, 6 years

If there has been a change in pattern during the course of the illness, this is best mentioned at the onset:

Headaches 6 years, worse 2 years.

When the patient complains of two or more varieties of headache these can be nominated separately at the onset and a line drawn down the middle of the history sheet so that data for each type of headache can be set out side by side. As an example let us take the history of a hypothetical woman aged 30 years, writing down the important positive and negative features in abbreviated form.

Headaches (1) unilateral with vomiting, 6 years;
(2) dull bilateral, 2 years.

The history may be written as follows:

	Type (1)	Type (2)
Frequency:	4 every month	almost daily
Duration	1 day	most of day
Site:	frontotemporal (L or R)	bifrontal
Quality:	throbbing, then severe and constant	dull, constant pressing
Time of onset:	any time, often 4–5 a.m.	on rising
Mode of onset:	occasionally blurred vision precedes headache by 10 min.	headache only
Associated features:	nausea, vomiting, photophobia, blurred vision, blood-shot eyes, no teichopsia no diplopia	light-headed at times no other symptoms

	no paraesthesiae no paresis no dysphasia slurred speech, vertigo and ataxia at height of headache lack of concentration no faintness, loss of consciousness polyuria as headache eases	
Precipitating factors:	attacks more frequent with menses alcohol, fatty foods, missing a meal may trigger attacks	worse during stress at work, entertaining at home, or when children misbehave
Relieving factors	no headache for last 6 months of her two pregnancies	no change during pregnancies
	frequency unaltered by vacations	eases when on vacation
	rest and darkness ergotamine tartrate, if taken at onset, shortens attack to 2 hours no trial of interval medication	relieved for 3 hours by A.P.C. powders improved by alcohol
Pattern	Migraine	Tension headache

A clinical pattern has thus emerged of a fairly constant tension headache, punctuated by frequent attacks of migraine. Such a history is not uncommon and is a cause of considerable disability. The combination of two types of headache must be recognized at the onset to guide the taking of the remainder of the history and to point the way to effective treatment. Once the pattern of headache is established, attention is turned to the general health of the patient, with specific enquiries about symptoms of conditions which may give rise to headache.

General health

It is important to determine at the outset whether headache is one facet of a systemic disease, or whether it may be regarded as an isolated problem.

The child who is failing to gain weight, does not look well, has altered in disposition and complains of headache, is a worrying problem. Cerebral tumour, tuberculous meningitis, and blood disorders such as leukaemia may first make themselves known in this way. In some illnesses of sudden onset, there may only be a vague malaise to indicate that headache is not primarily of intracranial origin; for example, acute nephritis can present with headache, hypertension and papilloedema without urinary symptoms. On the other hand, chronic infections, collagen diseases and endocrine disorders may all have caused an unmistakable deterioration in the patient's health before the development of headache.

At any age impairment of general health with loss of weight raises the possibility of malignant disease. In the group aged from 55 years onwards, general malaise, loss of weight, night sweats and aching of the joints and muscles should make one think of temporal arteritis as a source of headache.

System review

It is always helpful to ask leading questions concerning each bodily system at the conclusion of the history of the present illness. In a patient with headache, the eyes, ears, nose and throat, teeth and neck should be included in this review. The chronic obstruction of one or other nostril in vasomotor rhinitis or chronic respiratory tract infection may suggest the possibility of sinusitis. The eye may become proptosed with retro-orbital tumours or a mucocele projecting into the orbit from the frontal sinus. Dimness of vision and 'haloes' seen around lights may mark the onset of glaucoma. Complaints of impaired eyesight may draw attention to compression of the visual pathways. Papilloedema may be symptomless or the patient may notice blurring of vision on bending the head forwards. In contrast, visual loss is severe in retrobulbar neuritis and may be complete.

A space-occupying lesion or other intracranial disturbance such as progressive hydrocephalus becomes much more likely if the recent onset of headache is associated with any of the following symptoms:

Drowsiness at inappropriate times
Vomiting without apparent cause
Fits
Sudden falling attacks, in which consciousness may be retained
Progressive neurological deficit of any kind, for example, mental deterioration, impairment of senses of smell, vision or hearing. (It is remarkable how a unilateral nerve deafness may be present for years without being complained of, or even noticed, by the patient)

Double vision
Weakness or sensory impairment of the face or limbs on one or other
side
Disturbed co-ordination or loss of balance, with or without vertigo
Polyuria and polydipsia
Progressive change in pituitary function. Symptoms suggesting
hypopituitarism are asthenia, diminished libido, reduction of body
hair, lessened shaving frequency in men, premature cessation of
menstruation in women, the skin becoming soft and finely wrinkled
in both sexes, and the delay of pubescence in the child. On the other
hand hyperpituitarism may be responsible for excessive growth and
early pubescence in the young, and deepening of the voice, enlargement of the jaw and hands in adults.

Past health

A head injury at any time in the past 2 years may be of relevance.
Subdural haematoma may follow a blow on the head which the patient
considers trivial.

A number of episodes of 'encephalitis' or any severe headache with
neck stiffness should arouse suspicion of bleeding from a cerebral
angioma. A useful additional point in the history is the development of
nerve-root pains in the back, buttocks and thighs some hours or days
after the onset of headache, caused by blood tracking down the subarachnoid space to the cauda equina.

Any operations should be noted. The 'mole' removed 7 years ago
may be the secondary melanoma of today. A past tuberculous infection
may have been aroused from years of slumber.

Any debilitating illness or the use of corticosteroids may reactivate
tuberculous lesions or prepare the way for cryptococcal meningitis.
Recurrent renal infections or stones may underlie present hypertension.
Sinusitis and recurrent ear infections are of importance, particularly in
children.

Vomiting attacks and 'car sickness' in childhood commonly precede
migraine in later life. The author has always enquired after asthma, hay
fever, hives, eczema and other allergies in patients with migraine but
now doubts the relevance of these questions for reasons which will
become apparent in the chapter on migraine (*see Chapter 10*).

Family history

Both migraine and tension headache run in families but there is little
tendency for cluster headache to do so. Information may be gained

about a familiar proneness to malignancy, tuberculosis, hypertension and other disorders which may relate to the problem of headache.

Personal background

Occupation

The patient's occupation may have direct relevance to the problem of headache in the case of certain infections such as Q fever in abattoir workers. Exposure to toxic or vasodilator substances in some chemical processes, or the tedium of a repetitive job in a noisy environment, may be responsible for headache occurring at work. The patient's interest in his occupation may have been lost for a number of reasons, perhaps the inability to see the end-result of his labour, or from the pressure of uninspired or heavy-handed management. The levelling out in middle age, when a progress assessment shows that some dreams will never be fulfilled, may cause a reaction of anxiety and depression. The waning of old skills or the difficulty in accommodating to new ideas and techniques may cast gloom over the years before retirement and when retirement finally comes it may remove an important source of motivation and take much of the zest from life.

Personal or family problems

The possible psychological factors which may underlie the anxiety of a child, adolescent, unmarried adult or married couple are legion. Pressure on the individual to achieve a succession of goals now starts in primary school and the goals set by parents for their children are often quite unrealistic. Feelings of inadequacy and frustration are not uncommon as a result. Statisticians would be embarrassed if every child turned out to be of above-average intelligence, personality and sporting ability.

Parental separation or divorce, or a strained marriage continuing for the sake of the children, are common causes of insecurity, tension and behaviour disturbance in childhood. It requires patient and devoted team-work between husband and wife to bring up a family successfully at the best of times.

Sexual problems may be of importance at any age. The containment within accepted social bounds of the sexual vigour of youth and the maintenance of satisfactory sexual life in marriage during the mature middle years among the tensions of work and child-raising may each bring difficulties. The unmarried of any age may be troubled by the instability of their sexual and social relationships, with the spectre of loneliness at the end of the line.

All information volunteered about the patient's way of life should be considered, while bearing in mind that stress is usually insufficient in itself to cause headache. The problem lies more often in the failure of adjustment of a patient to a common situation which would not trouble most people.

Habits

The personal history also covers intake of alcohol, smoking habits and the consumption of headache powders and other drugs. The daily ingestion of up to 10 headache powders (usually containing aspirin, phenacetin and caffeine) by patients with tension headache is not uncommon and may alert the examiner to the possibility of methaemo-globinaemia or chronic renal disease from the long-continued use of analgesics. The author remembers one patient who nibbled 100 mg tablets of pentobarbitone throughout the day 'to steady the nerves', up to a total of 12 tablets daily. She would not divulge how she obtained such liberal supplies but her habituation was a psychiatric problem in its own right.

Some proprietary relaxing agents which can be bought from a pharmacist without a prescription contain a monureide and bromide. The development of bromism with headache and confusion may be insidious.

Certain foods may precipitate a headache in susceptible people. Many migraineurs blame fatty foods, chocolates and certain fruits, particularly oranges. An interesting form of headache has recently been described in patients who have eaten a Chinese meal when monosodium glutamate has been used liberally in the preparation of the food and this has been called the Chinese restaurant syndrome.

Red wines contain tyramine and histamine which may induce migraine or other vascular headaches in a dosage lower than that usually required to produce a 'hangover'. It is said that a chronic alcoholic rarely suffers from headache and that it is advisable to think of the possibility of a subdural haematoma if he does complain of recent headaches.

Emotional state

As the personal history is taken, some insight is usually gained into whether the patient's symptoms are exaggerated by loneliness and introspection or whether they are being played down by one who has an active and interesting life. The history is a second-hand experience which is coloured by the emotional expression of the person telling the story. While the history is being recorded it may be possible to discern whether the patient reacts to problems with physical manifestations of tension by frowning, clenching the jaws or holding the head and neck rigidly. It is important to look for symptoms of depression, such as loss of interest in work, homelife or personal affairs; or staying at home and not wanting to see friends or continue with previous activities. Depressive symptoms are most important to recognize since their treatment may play a big part in restoring pleasure to life, quite apart from relieving the headache which is often a reflection of the depressive state.

REFERENCES

Adams, F. (1841). *The Extant Works of Aretaeus, The Cappadocian,* p. 294. London: Sydenham Society

Critchley, M. (1967). Migraine from Cappadocia to Queen Square. In *Background to Migraine* p. 28, Ed. by R. Smith. London: Heinemann.

Stead, W. W., Heyman, A., Thompson, H.K., and Hammond, W.E. (1972). Computer-assisted interview of patients with functional headache. *Archs intern. Med.* **129,** 950

Four

Pattern Recognition from the History

The need for a careful and systematic history was presented in the previous chapter. The information about the headache obtained under each descriptive subheading is responsible for adding a valuable contribution to a differential diagnosis. The taking of a history is an active process. The enquiry after each aspect is like adding a chemical reagent to an unknown mixture and observing what takes place. Each step assists in the classification of headache and hence its identification.

Each subheading will be considered in turn to evaluate its significance in diagnosis or management of headache problems.

Length of illness

The length of time for which a patient has been troubled by headache is the first guide as to whether the symptom portends some malign or progressive neurological disorder which requires further investigation. At one end of the scale, the sudden onset of severe headache, possibly followed by impairment of consciousness or focal neurological signs, suggests some serious illness such as subarachnoid haemorrhage or meningitis. At the other end of the scale, a patient who has had headaches regularly for 20, 30 or 40 years is most likely to have some form of vascular headache (migraine or one of its variants), or chronic tension (muscle-contraction) headache. The first attack of migraine which a patient experiences may be confusing unless it is preceded by characteristic symptoms, and may suggest systemic infection, encephalitis or meningitis.

Between the very acute and very chronic headaches lie the most difficult to interpret, those which have developed over some days, weeks or months. The subacute headache may have a relatively simple explanation such as sinusitis or some ocular cause but one must be on guard against less common but more lethal conditions such as subdural haematoma, cerebral tumour or other causes of increased intracranial pressure, or, in the age group 55–70 years, the insidious onset of temporal (giant-cell) arteritis.

Frequency and duration of headache

These two parameters establish the temporal pattern which is so important in the diagnosis of recurrent headache. In this group the main conditions to be considered are migraine, cluster headache, trigeminal neuralgia (tic douloureux), tension and tension-vascular headache.

Migraine may recur irregularly at intervals of months or years but commonly a pattern has become established by the time a patient seeks medical advice. The headache may be linked to the menstrual cycle or may appear one to ten times each month without any obvious cause, disappearing only during pregnancy, holidays, admission to hospital or other periods of prolonged rest. It may last from a few hours to several days, but is usually followed by a period of freedom from headache before the next attack starts.

Cluster headache, on the other hand, has an intriguing periodicity. It usually recurs in bouts lasting from 2 weeks to 3 months and then vanishes completely for 3 months to as long as 4 years. During a bout, the headache returns once, twice or more in 24 hours, and lasts from 10 minutes to 2 hours on each occasion. The fact that the pain persists for this length of time clearly distinguishes it from trigeminal neuralgia, which recurs as transient jabs of pain, each lasting a fraction of a second, although the jabs may be repetitive. The two disorders are mentioned together because they are commonly confused in general practice. Many patients with cluster headache are referred with the provisional diagnosis of trigeminal neuralgia, probably because the pattern of cluster headache is not widely known. One point that the conditions have in common is the tendency to spontaneous remission for months or years. The distinction between the two is most important because the mechanism and treatment of each are entirely different.

Tension headache is set apart from those just considered by the absence of any paroxysmal quality or periodicity about its course. While acute forms of tension headache may appear at the end of a stressful day in a busy office or a household of screaming children, the usual story of the habitué is that there is always a headache lurking in the background. Such patients have some sort of headache all day and every day. They are never really free except for an hour or two after ingestion of their favourite caffeine-containing analgesic. There is a form of headache intermediate between this undulating pattern and the paroxysms of migraine. This is termed tension-vascular headache because surges of more severe throbbing headache become superimposed every few days or weeks on an otherwise monotonous background of constant discomfort.

Site

Headache is commonly bilateral except in migraine attacks (of which about two-thirds are one-sided), cluster headache and tic douloureux (which are almost always strictly unilateral), local changes in the eye, sinuses, skull or scalp, and expanding lesions of one cerebral hemisphere. An aneurysm of the internal carotid artery may cause pain behind one eye by enlarging without rupturing. Subarachnoid haemorrhage from aneurysm or angioma may start with local pain but headache usually becomes general in distribution and spreads to the back of the neck. Space-occupying lesions may cause unilateral pain by displacement of vessels, but headache becomes bilateral if CSF pathways are obstructed. The site of headache is not reliable as a means of localizing cerebral tumour.

The headache of internal carotid thrombosis is unilateral, whereas in vertebrobasilar insufficiency pain involves the occipital area bilaterally. Scalp vessels may be involved separately in temporal arteritis so that pain is limited to the distribution of a specific artery. Less commonly, migraine headache may be limited to a particular part of the vascular tree, giving rise to frontal, temporal or occipital pain, or even involving the internal maxillary and other branches of the external carotid system to produce facial pain known as 'lower half headache'. The pain of cluster headache characteristically involves the eye and frontal region on one side and may radiate down to the nostril and cheek of the same side, overlapping the distribution of 'lower half headache'. The pain of tic douloureux is felt in one or more of the divisions of the trigeminal nerve, but starts in the first division (eye and forehead) in only 5 per cent of cases.

Tension headache is usually bilateral, but may sometimes be one-sided owing to asymmetrical muscular-contraction, found particularly if there is associated imbalance of the bite. The pain of temporomandibular arthritis, resulting from an unbalanced or closed bite, may radiate in all directions from the joint in front of the ear, so that it involves much of the face and temple.

Quality

The most important distinction here is between pulsating or throbbing headache, indicating a vascular origin, and a constant ache. Migraine commonly starts as a dull headache, soon develops a throbbing quality which then becomes a constant severe pain, possibly as the arterial wall becomes oedematous and less easily distended with each pulse. The pain of cluster headache is described as deep, boring and intense. Tic douloureux is a shock-like transient stab of intense severity. Tension headache is usually dull, constant, tight, pressing or band-like. Certain embellishments of the history may indicate hysterical characteristics ('as though my skull were going to burst into a thousand fragments'), or an obsessional personality. One patient kept a daily chart of his headaches, plotted on a scale from H1 to H10 ('you can see where my headache went up to H9: that's almost as much as a body can bear'). The severity of headache is often a quality of diagnostic significance—the pain of cluster headache, tic douloureux and some attacks of migraine may indeed approach 'H9'.

Time of onset

Headaches resulting solely from hypertension, which are really quite uncommon, are present on waking but pass off as soon as the patient gets up and about. Migraine and tension-vascular headaches may also be present on waking or awaken the patient from sleep at 3 or 4 a.m. Cluster headache occurs by night as well as by day and frequently wakes the patient 1 or 2 hours after retiring. Tension headache does not wake the patient at night unless a vascular element becomes superimposed. The tense patient may or may not wake up free of headache but usually becomes aware of the familiar sensation as soon as the day's activities start.

The time of onset of headache is more important from the therapeutic than the diagnostic point of view. It is useless to prescribe ergotamine tartrate at the onset of a migraine attack if the patient's headache is in full bloom on waking. Medication has to be given the night before to anticipate the morning's episode. Similarly, an injection of ergotamine tartrate or an oral dose of methysergide is given on retiring to prevent nocturnal paroxysms of cluster headache.

Mode of onset

The only form of headache with a recognizable prodrome is migraine. For 10 to 40 minutes before the headache starts there may be visual hallucinations or a complex succession of neurological symptoms which adhere to much the same sequence on each occasion. Visual hallucinations may take the form of simple flashes of light or a coloured display of zig-zag scintillations (fortification spectra) moving slowly across the field leaving a scotoma behind. There may be patchy or generalized blurring of vision at the height of the disturbance or a clearly defined homonymous hemianopia.

Associated phenomena

There are a wide variety of symptoms linked with migraine headache, including photophobia, gastrointestinal disturbance, fluid retention, and focal neurological changes, which will be discussed in detail in Chapter 10.

The reddened forehead, injected conjunctiva, lacrimating eye and occasional Horner's syndrome of cluster headache are distinctive vascular phenomena. The nostril on the affected side may block or run with fluid.

The meningeal irritation of subarachnoid haemorrhage, meningitis and encephalitis causes a protective reflex muscle spasm of the extensor muscles of the neck which is manifest clinically as neck rigidity.

The sudden headache caused by a colloid cyst blocking the flow of CSF in the third ventricle may be accompanied by a 'drop attack', a sudden loss of power in the legs, caused by compression of the midline reticular formation. Consciousness is not necessarily lost with drop attacks. With any space-taking lesion, or progressive hydrocephalus, the patient may become drowsy, yawn frequently or vomit without preliminary nausea. Fits or other symptoms of focal cortical irritation may precede headache or appear as the headache intensifies. Diplopia may herald the onset of compression of the third cranial nerve, a sinister sign of an expanding intracranial mass forcing part of the temporal lobe downwards through the tentorial opening.

Rigors and sweats in any acute infectious process, nasal obstruction in sinusitis, conjunctival and circumcorneal injection in ocular conditions, are all indications of the source of headache.

Precipitating or aggravating factors

Any intracranial vascular headache, whether it be caused by 'hangover', hypoglycaemia or intracranial tumour, will be made worse by jarring, sudden movements of the head, coughing, sneezing or straining. 'Cough headache' is not always associated with intracranial tumour but can be benign, if unexplained, vascular syndrome in its own right. Bending the head forwards may bring on a severe paroxysmal headache in patients with colloid cyst of the third ventricle, or other forms of obstructive hydrocephalus.

Sensitivity to light is a common feature of diffuse intracranial disturbance such as meningitis or encephalitis as well as migraine. Glare, loud noises and even strong odours are liable to initiate or worsen tension headache as well as migraine.

Exercise aggravates vascular headache of any type and the occasional individual may suffer disability as a result of exercise alone. Sexual intercourse may bring on vascular or tension-vascular headaches and has been known to precipitate subarachnoid haemorrhage.

Some people are liable to a dull, vascular headache on missing a meal or several hours after a meal, and hypoglycaemia may provoke a migraine attack in susceptible patients. Certain foods are said to induce migraine. There is some evidence that ingestion of tyramine-containing foods may exert a chemical influence, but doubt has been cast on whether fatty foods, chocolates, oranges and other traditional migraine precipitants act specifically or by a psychological conditioning process. Vascular reactivity appears to be altered by hormonal changes, thus accounting for the association between migraine and menstruation, and its relief in some women during pregnancy.

Alcohol usually triggers cluster headache during a bout but not at other times. It may also bring on migraine when the patient is in a susceptible phase (not in the refractory period after an attack has recently ended) and some careful observers assure the author that red wines are much more liable to do this than white.

The explosive pains of tic douloureux may be detonated by stimulation of any area served by the trigeminal nerve. Talking, chewing, swallowing, shaving or even a puff of wind blowing on to the face are trigger factors commonly mentioned. Pain arising from the teeth is usually exacerbated by hot or cold fluids in the mouth. Movement of the jaw will add a sharp quality to the pain of temporomandibular arthritis.

Changes in barometric pressure may make the pain of sinusitis worse. Anyone who has ever had a cold when travelling by air and experienced pain from the sinuses during the descent will be sufficiently impressed to carry a nasal decongestant in future. Curiously, migraine may also follow sudden changes in barometric pressure, although the reason is unknown.

The relatively uncommon headache of cervical spondylosis is understandably aggravated by neck movement, just as the muscle-contraction headache of eyestrain is brought on by reading or close work. Tension headache may correlate fairly closely with periods of turbulence caused by worry, anger or excitement, but in the chronic form it may persist inexorably, no matter how calm the waters. Migraine may occur at a time of stress but it more commonly follows some hours after relaxation from stress or even the following day, as in 'weekend migraine'.

Relieving factors

Pressure on the distended scalp arteries, or over the common carotid artery of the affected side, and the use of hot or cold compresses, are often helpful in migraine. The migrainous patient usually prefers to lie in a darkened room whereas the sufferer from cluster headache prefers to sit up or pace the floor, holding his hand over the affected eye. Rebreathing into a paper bag or the inhalation of carbon dioxide 10 per cent in air or oxygen is said to shorten the vasoconstrictive phase of migraine.

Rest is usually essential to relieve intracranial vascular headache but the early morning headache of hypertension is improved by the upright position. Headache triggered by hypoglycaemia is not necessarily relieved by the taking of food.

The pain of sinusitis is abolished when the sinuses are cleared by the relief of nasal obstruction. The avoidance of chewing on one side and excessive jaw clenching eases the pain of temporomandibular strain or arthritis until dental attention can be obtained.

Voluntary relaxation of forehead and jaw muscles will reduce the severity of tension headache and the use of alcohol or other vasodilator substances such as nicotinic acid may temporarily abolish it.

Aspirin will stop the pain of migraine in childhood but not in adult life. Aspirin continues to be useful in other mild forms of head pain. In combination with phenacetin and caffeine as APC powders it forms part of the national diet for many, not only for patients with tension headache but also for those who think they might get a headache if they do not take these powders.

More specific methods of relieving headache will be discussed later in the appropriate chapters.

It is to be hoped that sufficient of the factors mentioned in this chapter will emerge during the taking of a clinical history to form a clear clinical impression of the headache pattern and an opinion about the group to which the headache belongs and its probable cause. Well-directed enquiries may bring out important points which the patient has neglected to mention. If the diagnosis is not evident after taking the clinical history, at least the physician should know what to look for on physical examination and should also have formed an opinion as to whether the headache warrants further investigation.

Five

Physical Examination

After hearing the patient's history, the physician may be alerted to look particularly carefully at certain aspects of the physical examination. In any event, the patient complaining of headache warrants a full examination. This will often be negative, but it is important to know that it is negative. The emphasis of examination will naturally be on the head and the nervous system, but there are so many ways in which headache may be produced that general examination must not be neglected.

General appearance

The general appearance of the patient often gives some clue about the nature of the headache. The transfer of a moist handkerchief from the palm of one hand to the other, the intertwining of the fingers, the restless movements and occasional sighing respiration are indications of nervous tension as valid as the furrowed brow and periodic thrusting forward or clenching of the jaw.

The shape of the face, the size of the jaw and hands, the texture of the skin and hair, and the timbre of the voice may direct attention to the endocrine system and to the pituitary gland in particular.

If a patient is seen while suffering from cluster headache, the forehead may be flushed and conjunctival vessels dilated only on the side of the headache. A partial Horner's syndrome may be present with drooping eyelid and small pupil, and tears may be observed running from the affected eye (*Figure 5.1*). In migraine, the patient is more often pale than flushed but the conjunctivae are nonetheless injected, more so on the side of the headache. Pulsation of the temporal vessels may be greater on the affected side and distended veins may be seen to arch

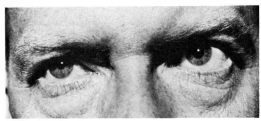

Figure 5.1. Paralysis of the ocular sympathetic nerve during an attack of cluster headache. The conjunctiva is injected on the affected side and a tear can be seen glistening in the conjunctival sac

across the forehead or temple. Thickened vessels may be visible in temporal arteritis.

The head may be held to one side, with the neck rotated, in some cases of posterior fossa tumour, resembling spasmodic torticollis in posture.

Mental state

The mental state of the patient will have been assessed superficially during history-taking. Drowsiness, confusion or disorientation may indicate a space-occupying lesion or diffuse cerebral disorder such as meningitis or encephalitis. There may be indications of a focal cortical lesion preventing normal appreciation of the body image or understanding of the written or spoken word, which might thus give a false impression of general intellectual deterioration. The patient may be unable to express himself in words, mime, or writing, or to calculate or perform routine tasks, or distinguish between right and left because of a lesion of the dominant hemisphere. If cortical function is intact, the emotional tone of the patient must be assessed and a state of agitation or depression recognized.

Speech

If the patient is dysphasic, a note must always be made as to whether he or she is right-or left-handed. The left hemisphere is almost invariably responsible for speech mechanisms in right-handed patients, but in left-handers dysphasia may result from lesions in either hemisphere.

Skull

The skull must always be examined in patients with headache. This may seem self-evident but is often forgotten. A search of the scalp may disclose local infection, bone tumour or the hardened tender arteries of temporal arteritis (*see Figure 6.1*). The bones may be sensitive to percussion overlying inflamed sinuses or mastoid processes. The fontanelles should be palpated in infants since bulging of the fontanelles is a direct indication of increased intracranial pressure. It is worthwhile measuring the head circumference in a child at its widest point since repeated measurements are of value in detecting progressive hydrocephalus.

A short neck makes one think of congenital platybasia which may cause a slowly progressive hydrocephalus.

Auscultation of the skull (listening over the orbits, temples and mastoid processes) may disclose a systolic bruit in the case of aneurysm, angioma, vascular tumours or stenosis of the cranial vessels. When the examiner is listening over the closed eyelids, the patient is requested to open the other eye and hold the breath to prevent eyelid flutter and breath sounds from obscuring a bruit. Skull bruits are often normal in children under the age of 10 years and may be discounted unless loud and unilateral. An unexpected dividend from auscultation of the skull is that the sound of muscle contraction may be heard over the temporal and frontal muscles in patients who are unable to relax. Detecting this constant noise of muscle fibres straining one against the other makes one aware of nervous tension which might previously have been concealed.

Spine

The cervical spine is tested for tenderness and mobility. Resistance of the neck to passive flexion and Kernig's sign are usually present in meningeal irritation.

Gait and stance

An unsteady wide-based gait may be observed as a result of cerebellar disturbance. It may indeed be the only sign of a midline cerebellar lesion in the early stages. The author recalls a one-legged man who suddenly lost the ability to walk with a crutch. There was no evidence of a cerebellar lesion other than his one-legged ataxia. Subsequent events disclosed a secondary carcinoma from the lung in the vermis of the cerebellum.

Special senses

Smell

The nostrils are often blocked in rhinitis and sinusitis so that the sense of smell cannot be adequately assessed. The sense of smell may be lost when the olfactory nerve is damaged by head injury or by a tumour in the vicinity of the olfactory groove. The sense of smell should always be tested when a patient's intellectual ability has deteriorated since a frontotemporal tumour may cause both anosmia and mental confusion.

Vision

Circumcorneal injection may be observed in acute glaucoma and increased intra-ocular pressure may give rise to a palpable firmness of the eye. The significance of changes in visual acuity, visual fields and optic fundi is too large a subject to be encompassed here. It is sufficient to say that the visual fields of every patient complaining of a headache which does not conform to a typical benign pattern should be tested to confrontation and the optic fundi should always be examined.

The most common question to be decided is the presence or absence of papilloedema. Swelling of the optic disc usually starts at the poles and spreads to the nasal aspect of the disc before the temporal margin. The optic cup becomes filled-in and pulsation of veins where they cross over the rim of the optic cup can no longer be seen. If, after careful examination by an ophthalmologist, there is any dispute about whether an unusual appearance of the optic discs could be one of the forms of congenital pseudopapilloedema, the matter can be settled by fundus photography after the injection of fluorescein.

Swelling of the optic disc in optic (retrobulbar) neuritis is called papillitis and the appearance may be indistinguishable from papilloedema. Unlike papilloedema, papillitis causes severe impairment of vision. There is only slight restriction of the peripheral visual fields in papilloedema and the blind spot enlarges as swelling of the disc increases, since the blind spot is the projection of the optic disc in the visual fields.

Optic atrophy may result from interference with the blood supply to the optic nerve, long-standing papilloedema, retrobulbar neuritis or compression of the optic nerve or the optic chiasm. Occasionally a lesion behind the eye such as meningioma growing from the sphenoid wing compresses one optic nerve and its surrounding subarachnoid space, and then expands sufficiently to increase intracranial pressure or to impair venous return from the other eye so that papilloedema develops on the side opposite to the origin of the lesion. This combination of optic atrophy in one eye and papilloedema in the other is known as the Foster Kennedy syndrome.

Sybhyaloid haemorrhages may be observed after subarachnoid bleeding, and perivascular nodules may rarely be seen in tuberculous meningitis or disseminated lupus erythematosus. Circumscribed areas of choroidal atrophy may be a sign of toxoplasmosis.

Hearing

The eardrums should be inspected, particularly in children, since otitis media may spread centrally to cause thrombosis of the lateral sinus (otitic hydrocephalus) or to form an abscess of temporal lobe or cerebellum. Conduction deafness is demonstrated by tuning fork tests in the case of otitis media or Eustachian catarrh. A unilateral nerve deafness should be further investigated by audiometry, loudness-balance tests, caloric responses, radiography of the petrous temporal bone, and possibly tomography or posterior fossa myelography, to ensure that an acoustic neurinoma is not missed.

Other cranial nerves

A latent ocular imbalance may be unmasked by any infectious or debilitating illness and give rise to diplopia which may be misinterpreted as indicating a paresis of one or other of the extra-ocular muscles. A sixth nerve palsy may be found on the side of a lateral sinus thrombosis, and bilateral sixth nerve palsies may be found with any case of acute hydrocephalus or cerebral oedema because the sixth nerves are compressed in their long intracranial course by the expanded brain.

Progressive enlargement of the pupil on one side, with or without other signs of a third nerve palsy, is an indication for immediate action since the third nerve may be compressed by any expanding lesion forcing the uncus and medial aspect of the temporal lobe downwards through the tentorial opening into the posterior fossa. It can be taken as a rule that the dilated pupil is always on the side of the expanding lesion (such as a subdural haematoma) and exceptions to this rule are rare indeed. Inability to elevate both eyes is a sign of compression of the midbrain (Parinaud's syndrome) but it should be remembered that many elderly patients have difficulty in elevating the eyes.

The sudden onset of a third nerve palsy with pain behind the eye is most frequently caused by the sudden enlargement of an aneurysm (*see Figure 8.1*), although this may also occur in the rare syndrome of ophthalmoplegic migraine.

If the patient's consciousness becomes impaired so that voluntary eye movements are no longer possible, the integrity of the third, fourth and sixth nerves may be tested by the 'doll's eyes manoeuvre'. When the head is rotated to one side, the eyes roll to the opposite side, thus producing the movements of lateral conjugate deviation. Similarly, if the chin is pushed down on the chest the eyes elevate and if the head is extended the eyes roll downwards.

The presence of Horner's syndrome in cluster headache has already been mentioned, and it may also be seen occasionally in migraine. The pupil of one side may remain small between paroxysms of cluster headache or after a severe attack of migraine. Both pupils may be small in a pontine lesion.

Any cranial nerve may be involved by direct compression. It is particularly important to test facial sensation carefully, including 2-point discrimination on the lip, and to check the corneal responses in patients with trigeminal neuralgia. If there is any sensory deficit the patient must be suspected of having a lesion compressing the trigeminal nerve or a pontine plaque of multiple sclerosis.

If corticobulbar pathways are involved, weakness of the lower face will be detected and the jaw jerk and facial reflexes may increase. A bifrontal lesion will result in a pouting of the lips on tapping in the midline between the nose and mouth.

Motor system

Signs of an upper motor neurone or cerebellar disturbance may be detected with an expanding intracranial lesion. When the patient's arms are extended and the eyes are closed, the arm may slowly fall away on the affected side. With an upper motor neurone (pyramidal) lesion, muscle tone may be increased and movements of the fingers become slow and clumsy. Power is reduced, particularly in the extensor and abductor groups of the upper limbs and flexors of the lower limbs. This distribution of weakness is characteristic of an upper motor neurone lesion, whether or not the deep reflexes are increased or the plantar response is extensor on that side.

A hemiparesis is most commonly found on the side opposite to a cerebral lesion but in a minority of patients with a rapidly expanding mass, such as subdural haematoma, the hemiparesis is found on the same side as the lesion. The reason for this is that the growing mass pushes the midbrain over on to the tentorial edge so that the opposite cerebral peduncle is compressed. Since the pyramidal tracts cross below this level, the hemiparesis is on the same side as the causative lesion. Bilateral upper motor neurone signs may result from midbrain compression. A grasp reflex indicates a lesion of the opposite frontal lobe. An interesting sign, known as the palmar-mental response, may be elicited in patients with frontal lobe lesions. Stroking the thenar eminence firmly evokes a brief contraction of the muscles of the chin on the same side.

With a cerebellar lesion, the affected side is hypotonic. When the elbows are resting on a table with forearms vertical and wrist muscles relaxed, the hand hangs lower on the affected side. If the eyes are closed and the arms are lifted suddenly to a point at right angles to the body the arm on the affected side overshoots and oscillates. The knee jerk is pendular on the affected side. Rapid and alternating movements are impaired and finger—nose and heel—shin co-ordination is defective. The gait is wide-based and halting, and the patient turns jerkily 'by numbers' and tends to stumble to the side of the lesion.

Sensory system

A parietal lobe disturbance may cause subtle sensory deficit with difficulty in discriminating two points or recognizing objects placed in the hand. Sensory inattention should be sought by touching both arms or legs simultaneously with the patient's eyes closed. Long sensory tracts may be involved with deeply-placed cerebral lesions or brainstem disorders, resulting in a more clear-cut sensory disturbance.

Sphincters and sexual functions

Urgency of micturition may appear with upper motor neurone lesions, and a casual approach towards the time and place of relaxing the sphincters may be a feature of frontal lobe disturbance. Impotence can result from a temporal lobe lesion. The author recently saw a woman with a frontal lobe tumour present with urinary incontinence while her intellect was sufficiently preserved for her to be distressed by the trail she left behind her.

General examination

The presence of brownish patches in the skin (*café au lait* patches) with or without cutaneous neurofibromas indicates that the patient has a greater chance than the average of harbouring an intracranial tumour or phaeochromocytoma. Not only neurofibromas but also meningiomas and gliomas are more common in neurofibromatosis or its formes frustes. The observation of cutaneous angiomas raises the possibility of an intracerebral angioma. Peutz—Jeghers syndrome is an unusual familial condition characterized by dark pigmentation on the lips and buccal mucosa which is associated with polyposis of the small intestine. There may be an increased tendency to intracranial tumour in this condition as there is in polyposis coli, since I have seen such a patient with multiple intracranial meningiomas.

Smoothness of the skin, paucity of body hair and testicular atrophy should be look for as signs of pituitary deficiency.

Any scar in the skin warrants an enquiry about the nature of the lesion removed, as melanoma is notorious for presenting with metastases in the nervous system years after the primary tumour has been removed. Skin rashes are of importance in many infectious processes, such as meningococcaemia, glandular fever and the exanthemata associated with headache.

The association of a thin build with long fingers and toes and a high arched palate, known as Marfan's syndrome, carries an increased liability to intracranial aneuryms. Other inconstant features include hypertension from coarctation of the aorta, congenital heart defects and congenital dislocation of the lenses of the eye, which transmits a noticeable quivering movement to the iris on sudden eye movements.

Enlargement of lymph glands and spleen is related to the problem of headache in glandular fever, blood dyscrasias and the reticuloses. Ecchymoses and purpura may be observed in thrombocytopenic purpura with neurological complications.

Urine-testing does not contribute to the solution of most headache problems but the presence of albuminuria may be relevant to some causes of headache. The finding of a cardiac valvular defect should suggest the possibility of cerebral emboli (from atrial clot or subacute bacterial endocarditis) where transient cerebral episodes and headache are of recent onset.

Since most systemic disorders may have a neurological component, and most cerebral disorders may have headache as a symptom, there is no need to catalogue all the possible signs which could be unearthed by careful examination which may bear direct relevance to the problem of headache. Having said this, it must be added that the majority of patients complaining of chronic headache do not have physical signs which pertain to their main symptom, unless we include constant muscular overactivity, the inability to relax, which is dealt with elsewhere. A number of other minor problems which require attention may be disclosed by a careful examination; many of them may have been a source of worry to the patient although unmentioned in the original history. There is no better start to the reassurance of a patient than the knowledge that a proper physical examination has been carried out as part of a careful clinical assessment.

Six

Pain from the Cranium, Cranial Nerves and Extracranial Structures

THE CRANIUM

It is remarkably uncommon to find a source of headache within the cranial bones, although some examples will be cited later of inflammatory or neoplastic lesions involving the sinuses or petrous temporal bones. Nevertheless it is always advisable to run one's hands over the scalp of anyone complaining of headache. Occasionally a scalp infection may give rise to pain which is described as headache. Any expanding lesion of bone which stretches the periosteum may cause local pain. Paget's disease of the skull may be associated with a vascular headache fluctuating in intensity, probably caused by increased cranial blood flow. The scalp may feel warm in Paget's disease because of arterio-venous shunting which may reach such proportions that cardiac output is substantially increased. The softening of bone in Paget's disease may cause the base of the skull to be invaginated by the atlas and axis, giving rise to 'basilar impression' (platybasia). In this condition the posterior fossa is distorted and the flow of CSF may be impaired with increase in intracranial pressure as described in Chapter 8 (*see Figure 8.8*).

INFLAMMATION OF EXTRACRANIAL ARTERIES

Systemic lupus erythematosus may be associated with headache and papilloedema which responds to corticosteroid administration

(Silberberg and Laties, 1973). In the absence of other neurological symptoms and signs, the presence of headache in this condition does not indicate involvement of the central nervous system (Atkinson and Appenzeller, 1975), presumably because the disease affects small blood vessels. By way of contrast, a related disorder, known as temporal or giant-cell arteritis has headache as its most important presenting symptom.

Temporal arteritis

Temporal arteritis affects women more than men in the ratio 7:4, mostly over the age of 50 years although one patient aged 35 years has been reported. Symptoms of systemic disturbance, such as loss of weight, night sweats, aching of joints and a low grade fever are commonly associated, thus merging into the syndrome known as 'polymyalgia rheumatica' (Hunder and Allen, 1974). Of 53 cases of temporal arteritis reported by Wadman and Werner (1972), 12 had a past history suggestive of rheumatoid arthritis and more than half complained of myalgic pains.

The majority of patients complain of head pains or headache, unilateral or bilateral, which may be localized to the affected scalp vessels. Pain in the jaw muscles on chewing is a pathognomonic symptom when it occurs, caused by intermittent claudication of the masseter from narrowing of the extracranial arteries. The disorder may also involve intracranial vessels, particularly the ophthalmic artery, causing blindness from retinal ischaemia and subsequent optic atrophy. The aorta, coronary, renal and iliac arteries have been implicated in some reported cases.

Typical temporal arteritis starts with pain over the affected scalp arteries which become thickened and cease to pulsate (*Figure 6.1*). They are usually tender when touched and the skin overlying them may become red. Paulley and Hughes (1960) summarized previous reports and added 76 cases of their own. They described atypical modes of presentation with facial neuralgia, mental changes, visual disturbance, cardiac ischaemia, 'anarthritic rheumatism, ear pains, vertigo and deafness, vomiting, meningeal irritation and pyrexia of unknown origin. Vision is lost in one or both eyes in about 20 per cent of untreated cases. One patient of mine, a wise old dairy farmer, virtually made his own diagnosis when he told me that the pulse in his right temple had stopped shortly before he lost his sight in the right eye.

Apart from obvious changes in the scalp vessels, the physical signs vary according to the extent of involvement of the cerebral and other

arteries. The ophthalmoscopic picture of central retinal artery thrombosis may be seen, retinal ischaemia and oedema with dimpling in the
macular region producing a greyish-red spot. At a later stage the optic
disc becomes atrophic.

The erythrocyte sedimentation rate (ESR) is greater than 45 mm/h in
most patients and ranges up to 120 mm/h. Electrophoresis of
serum proteins demonstrates increase in alpha- and beta-globulin

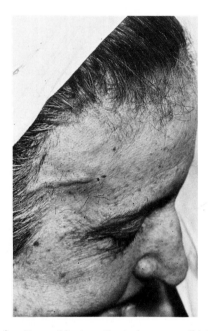

Figure 6.1. The characteristic appearance of temporal arteritis

fractions. Most patients have a mild hypochromic anaemia and polymorphonuclear leucocytosis. Biopsy of the temporal artery (or the
facial artery if this is more appropriate to the site of pain) shows
thickening of the intima, fibrosis and cellular infiltration of the vessel
wall, often with giant cells resembling those of tuberculous disease or
sarcoidosis, and thrombus formation in the lumen (*see Figure 6.2*). The
distribution of vascular changes may be patchy so that a negative
biopsy does not necessarily negate the diagnosis. Arteriography of the
external carotid circulation (Gillanders, Strachan and Blair, 1969) has
recently been used to indicate the sites most severely involved so that
an arterial biopsy may be selective.

The use of adrenal corticosteroids rapidly stops the pain and malaise
of the syndrome and it is generally accepted that the risk of ophthalmic

artery involvement is reduced to about half, but not completely obviated, by the use of steroids. Prednisone may be started in the dose of 40–60 mg daily and reduced slowly after some weeks to a maintenance dosage of 10–20 mg daily. Treatment may have to be continued for twelve months or more as relapse may take place if the patient is weaned off corticosteroids prematurely. The ESR and white cell count return to normal limits as the inflammation subsides with the use of steroids.

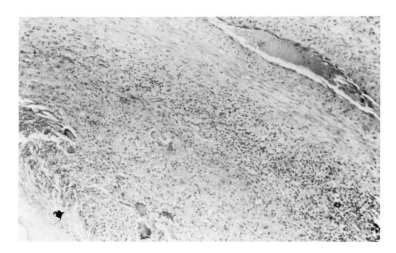

Figure 6.2. The biopsy of the vessel shown in Figure 6.1. The arterial wall is thickened with round cell infiltration and giant-cell formation

Early diagnosis is of great importance. A most tragic example of a missed opportunity was a patient whom I saw when she was totally blind. She had consulted her medical practitioner six months previously for generalized muscular aching, and she had noted pain in the jaws on chewing at that time. A blood count was done, but not an ESR. She was treated with a series of antirheumatic drugs without relief until she went blind in one eye. She was admitted to hospital where steroid treatment was started immediately but the next day she lost her vision in the other eye.

When the condition is suspected on the clinical history, whether or not the ESR is elevated, it is a good policy to have one temporal artery biopsied. Treatment can be started immediately, before the biopsy is taken. Steroid therapy may have to be continued for years and it is reassuring to have a firm histological diagnosis at the outset.

CAROTIDYNIA

There appear to be at least two varieties of carotidynia, a syndrome of neck pain associated with tenderness of the carotid artery (Roseman, 1968). One form is of acute onset in young or middle-aged adults in which the pain persists for an average of 11 days and does not usually recur. The pain radiates to the side of the face in about half the cases. Tenderness is maximal over the carotid bifurcation. There are usually no signs of systemic infection although some patients feel unwell and complain of nasal blockage and lacrimation. The ESR remains normal. The cause is unknown but the short course of the disorder suggests a viral infection. Treatment is symptomatic with analgesics. Prednisolone therapy has not proven helpful.

The other form of carotidynia may appear at any stage of adult life and recurs in attacks lasting minutes to hours, daily or weekly, often in conjunction with throbbing headache (Raskin and Prusiner, 1977). This form responds to ergotamine or substances such as methysergide used in the prophylaxis of migraine. Tenderness of the carotid artery is not uncommon in migraine and carotidynia may be an extreme form of this vascular sensitivity. Carotidynia has also been reported with temporal arteritis, fibrosis around the carotid sheath, and other conditions (Roseman, 1968).

PAIN FROM THE CRANIAL NERVES

Pain is referred to the head or face by any disturbance of the trigeminal nerve, and deep to the angle of the jaw, one side of the throat and tongue, by irritation of the glossopharyngeal nerve. The vagus and nervus intermedius of the facial nerve can refer pain to the ear. It is theoretically possible for the nervus intermedius and vagus nerves to refer pain to the posterior half of the head as discussed in Chapter 1.

Physiological stimulation

Excitation of the peripheral branches of cranial nerves by physiological stimuli may give rise to pain. Wearing a tight hat or headband may cause headache. Exposure to a cold wind or swimming in cold water may provoke headache, particularly sudden and severe if the unsuspecting subject dives into cold water. Another example, familiar to many, is 'ice-cream headache'.

Ice-cream headache

Holding ice or ice-cream in the mouth or swallowing it as a bolus may cause local pain in the palate or throat. It may also refer pain to the forehead or temple via the trigeminal nerve, and to the ear through the vagus nerve. The cause is sudden cooling of the mouth or pharynx, since cooling of the oesophagus or the stomach itself does not produce headache. Raskin (1976) found that 31 per cent of a non-migrainous group of patients had experienced ice-cream headache, compared with 93 per cent of a migrainous group. The headache in the migraine patients was more severe than in the control group.

Compression of cranial nerves

The first division of the trigeminal nerve may be compressed in the orbit, the superior orbital fissure, cavernous sinus or near the apex of the petrous temporal bone. Tumours such as a meningioma growing from the sphenoid wing or a pituitary tumour may refer pain to the forehead associated with diminished sensibility over the area supplied by the first division of the trigeminal nerve. The sudden onset of severe pain behind and above one eye may indicate the enlargement of an aneurysm of the internal carotid or posterior communicating artery (*see Figure 8.1*). The Gasserian ganglion may also be compressed by meningioma. A neuroma may arise from the fifth nerve. Trigeminal nerve compression is often painless but when pain is present it is usually constant and associated with sensory impairment in the appropriate distribution.

Tolosa-Hunt syndrome

Granulomatous tissue may ensheath the first division of the fifth cranial nerve as well as the third, fourth and sixth nerves in the vicinity of the superior orbital fissure. It causes a recurrent ophthalmoplegia which may be accompanied by pain behind and above the eye. Spontaneous remissions occur but the condition resolves rapidly with the use of corticosteroids. The aetiology is unknown.

Raeder's paratrigeminal neuralgia

This condition is a combination of pain of trigeminal distribution, usually over the forehead, with an ocular sympathetic paralysis (ptosis, miosis but sparing of sweating over the forehead) (Toussaint, 1968). This partial Horner's syndrome indicates a lesion of the sympathetic nerves in the wall of the internal carotid artery or orbit since those fibres responsible for sweating of the face travel with the external carotid artery and its branches. Raeder's syndrome was originally described in a patient with a meningioma between the internal carotid artery and Gasserian ganglion. It has also been reported following trauma, in which case there may have been a dissection or other damage to the wall of the internal carotid artery. Many of the reported cases cannot be distinguished from cluster headache (migrainous neuralgia), which is often accompanied by ptosis and miosis. Raeder's syndrome cannot therefore be regarded as an entity but serves to draw attention to the internal carotid artery in searching for its various causes.

Gradenigo's syndrome

Lesions of the apex of the petrous temporal bone cause pain referred to the frontotemporal region and ear in conjunction with a paralysis of the sixth cranial nerve which runs across the bone at that point. Gradenigo's syndrome was originally described as a complication of middle ear infections but may also be found with tumours arising from or invading this area (*see Figure 6.6*).

Postherpetic neuralgia

The Gasserian ganglion is affected in approximately 1 in 8 of patients with herpes zoster, and in four-fifths of these the ophthalmic division is singled out. The rash may also involve the external auditory meatus, the soft palate or the area supplied by the upper cervical roots. Paralysis of the third, fourth or sixth cranial nerves, or a facial palsy may accompany the herpetic eruption. The combination of a herpetic rash in the external auditory canal and a facial palsy results from invasion of the geniculate ganglion and is known as Ramsay Hunt syndrome. An unpleasant burning pain precedes the skin eruption by 2 to 4 days and persists in the partially anaesthetic area after the rash has subsided in about 10 per cent of cases. Pain in the distribution of the first division of the trigeminal nerve may cause diagnostic difficulties when it appears several days before the rash or, on rare occasions, without any rash at all.

Postherpetic neuralgia afflicts 30 per cent of patients over the age of 40 years who have suffered shingles, and 50 per cent of patients over the age of 60. Why the incidence increases with advancing years is unknown. In a review of the gate-control theory of pain, Nathan (1976) summarizes the conflicting views expressed in various reports of the pathological changes wrought by herpes zoster, concluding that the condition cannot be explained by the selective fall-out of a certain range of nerve fibres. Skin and nerve are involved by fibrous tissue with degeneration of large fibres followed by smaller fibres. The genesis of the pain is presumably related to a disturbance in the pattern of afferent impulses and the removal of some central inhibitory influence since pain usually persists after section of the trigeminal nerve or medullary tractotomy. The descending tract of the trigeminal nerve is the direct rostral continuation of the tract of Lissauer in the spinal cord. Like the tract of Lissauer, the ventrolateral portion of the descending trigeminal tract exerts a suppressor effect on sensory transmission in its neighbouring segments, and the dorsomedial portion has a facilitatory effect (Denny-Brown and Yanagisawa, 1973). Fibres from the ophthalmic division of the trigeminal nerve lie in the ventrolateral segment so that it is conceivable that the virus of herpes zoster could selectively damage this inhibitory area, thus permitting unrestrained onflow of afferent impulses responsible for postherpetic neuralgia.

The most satisfactory treatment of postherpetic neuralgia is its prevention by the use of steroids in the acute phase of the illness. Elliott (1964) summarized previous reports on steroid treatment and added 11 cases of his own in whom the pain cleared in an average of 3½ days after the start of treatment compared with 3½ weeks in those members of a control group who lost their pain spontaneously. Two of the control group developed persistent postherpetic neuralgia. Elliott quoted the experience of Scheie with more than 70 cases of herpes ophthalmicus in whom the pain was rapidly relieved by the use of steroids without any dissemination of the rash. The incidence of keratitis, uveitis and secondary glaucoma was reduced. The course of steroids should begin as soon as possible in the illness and comprises 60 mg of prednisone daily for one week, 30 mg daily for the second week and 15 mg daily for a third week. There have been reports of a generalized rash resembling chickenpox in some patients treated with steroids but the only serious or fatal complications have occurred in those whose immune mechanisms have been depleted by leukaemia or similar serious disorders.

Once postherpetic neuralgia is established I have found only two methods of treatment to be useful. The tricyclic antidepressant drugs, particularly amitriptyline, exert a pain-suppressing action and usually reduce the pain to a tolerable level. The dose can be started as 25 mg at night and gradually increased to 75 mg each night if the patient is not troubled by side-effects. Occasionally the dose may have to be increased to 150 mg daily. Amitriptyline therapy can be continued indefinitely if it is successful. Shanbrom (1961) reported that an intravenous drip of 500 ml procaine 0.1–0.2 per cent repeated up to 10 times if necessary relieved 13 out of 16 patients. I have used a xylocaine drip, 1 g of xylocaine being added to 500 ml of 5% glucose in N/5 saline and administered at the rate of 2mg/min (1 ml/min) as in the treatment of patients with cardiac dysrhythmias after myocardial infarction. This drip may be repeated 3 times or more. Diminution of postherpetic pain usually outlasts the duration of the infusion and is often permanent.

Central lesions

Estimates of the frequency with which trigeminal neuralgia occurs in multiple sclerosis vary from 1 to 8 per cent (Selby, 1975). From the other point of view, about 2 per cent of patients with trigeminal neuralgia have multiple sclerosis. In 80 to 90 percent of the documented cases, other symptoms of multiple sclerosis preceded the onset of trigeminal neuralgia by 1 to 29 years. In the remainder the facial pain was the presenting symptom and other signs of multiple sclerosis followed one month to six years later. Of patients with multiple sclerosis and trigeminal neuralgia, the pain becomes bilateral in 11 to 14 per cent compared with 3 to 5 per cent of patients with the idiopathic form. The pain is caused by a plaque of multiple sclerosis in the pons at the entry zone of the trigeminal nerve. Jannetta (1973) observed such plaques in 4 per cent of patients subjected to posterior fossa exploration for trigeminal neuralgia. Watkins and Espir (1969) reported that migrainous headache was more common in patients with multiple sclerosis, affecting 27 per cent of patients compared with 12 per cent of a control group. This association is difficult to explain and remains to be confirmed.

Central lesions other than multiple sclerosis rarely present with facial pain as an important symptom although unpleasant burning sensations may accompany any disturbance of the descending spinal tract of the fifth nerve or the spinothalamic tracts by glioma, syringomyelia or vascular disease. Diminution of sensibility to pinprick and temperature can usually be detected over the painful areas and the corneal response may be depressed.

Trigeminal neuralgia

The prevalence of trigeminal neuralgia has been estimated as 155 per million population (Selby, 1975). It affects women more than men in the ratio of 1.6:1. Its alternative name 'tic douloureux' (a painful spasm) came into use in the mid-eighteenth-century. The onset of the disorder is usually over the age of 40 years, with a mean age varying from 50 to 58 years in different reported series. Familial occurrence is rare.

The pain is strictly limited to some part of the distribution of the trigeminal nerve, involving the right side more than the left in the ratio 3:2. It usually starts in the second or third divisions, affecting the cheek or chin. Less than 5 per cent start in the first division. All 3 divisions have been involved in 10 to 15 per cent of reported cases, and the pain has become bilateral in 3 to 5 per cent. The pain is sudden, intense and stabbing in quality, lasting only momentarily but often recurring in repeated paroxysms. The patient can always identify trigger factors such as talking, chewing, swallowing, or touching the face or gums as in shaving or cleaning the teeth. There may also be trigger points, areas around the nose or lips, which are particularly liable to evoke a paroxysm if touched, the pain commonly being in the same division as the trigger point. The pain may recur daily for weeks or months and then remit for a period of time, even for years, before returning. This periodicity sometimes leads to confusion between tic douloureux and that other enigmatic, intermittent facial and head pain, cluster headache. There have indeed been reported instances of the two conditions being associated but this is rare and the characteristic lancinating pain of tic bears little resemblance to the boring pain of cluster headache which lasts for 10 minutes or more each time. Tic douloureux may occasionally occur with glossopharyngeal neuralgia so that pain is referred to the ear and throat as well as the trigeminal distribution. There is a tendency for tic douloureux to become progressively worse in frequency and severity of episodes. There is no sensory loss in idiopathic tic so that other conditions such as nerve compression or multiple sclerosis must be considered if sensation is found to be impaired.

Pathological changes noted in the Gasserian ganglion or trigeminal pathways are difficult to distinguish from age changes. The cause of the pain remains uncertain, whether mechanical compression or degenerative changes of the nerve initiate synchronous afferent volleys. It has been postulated that the condition may result from herpes simplex infection, from compression of the second and third divisions by the internal carotid artery, or from compression of the nerve by arterial loops at the point where it enters the pons.

The pain usually responds to the administration of carbamazepine (Tegretol) 200 mg three times daily, increasing to 400 mg three times daily if necessary (and if the patient is able to tolerate this dosage without giddiness and ataxia). Clonazepam (Rivotril, Clonopin) 2 mg three times daily has also been reported to control tic douloureux. Phenytoin (Dilantin) is rather less successful. The rationale for the use of these anticonvulsant drugs is that trigeminal neuralgia may be regarded as a 'peripheral epilepsy' caused by synchronous and often repetitive discharge of the sensory neurones of the trigeminal nerve or their central connections. Cabamazepine may cause leucopenia. For this reason patients should be warned to report for a blood count should they develop any infection. The blood may be checked every three months as a routine but it is doubtful whether regular blood counts really fulfil any useful function since leucopenia may appear quite suddenly. Carbamazepine may be used to tide the patient over a bout of trigeminal neuralgia and then withdrawn during a period of remission.

If the condition persists in spite of medical treatment, a surgical approach becomes necessary. Operations have been devised to decompress the Gasserian ganglion or sensory root with temporary relief or to compress these structures with more lasting relief, but alcohol injection or section of the sensory root have remained the standard surgical procedures. More recently, controlled thermocoagulation of the Gasserian ganglion by a probe inserted in the same manner as for alcohol injection, has provided relief of pain with little or no sensory impairment (Sweet and Wepsic, 1974). The technique offers hope of sparing the corneal reflex and thus preventing ocular complications. Jannetta (1973) advocates posterior fossa exploration, using a binocular microscope to examine the nerve at the point of entry into the pons. Of his first 100 patients, 94 were found to have some identifiable source of compression or irritation of the nerve fibres, usually by the superior cerebellar artery (85 patients). The anterior inferior cerebellar artery was responsible in 3 cases, a vein in 1, arteriovenous malformations in 2 and small tumours in 3 instances (acoustic neurinoma, meningioma and pontine glioma). In 4 patients, plaques of multiple sclerosis were observed and 2 had atrophic nerves. The arterial loops appeared to result from elongation of the vessels as a part of the ageing process. Removal of the loops from the nerve resulted in cure of the pain in 16 out of 17 cases. These observations have been dealt with in some detail since they place a new emphasis on the possible genesis and management of tic douloureux.

Glossopharyngeal neuralgia

Glossopharyngeal neuralgia is about 100 times less common than trigeminal neuralgia and causes a similar type of lancinating pain in the ear, base of the tongue, tonsillar fossa, or beneath the angle of the jaw (Chawla and Falconer, 1967). The distribution is not only in the sensory area of the glossopharyngeal nerve but also of the auricular and pharyngeal branches of the vagus nerve. It is provoked by swallowing, talking or coughing. If the pain does not respond to carbamazepine, intracranial section of the glossopharyngeal nerve and the upper two rootlets of the vagus nerve has been recommended.

Atypical facial pain

Depressed or anxious patients may present with a constant aching pain in the face which defies analysis, and does not respond to conventional headache remedies, or even to blockade or section of what would appear to be the appropriate cranial nerves. It could be said that it bears the same relationship to 'lower half headache' as tension headache does to migraine. The pain is commonly unilateral and is felt deeply in the angle of the nose or in the cheek. It is constant and boring in quality and may spread diffusely to other areas of the head or neck at times of exacerbation. There is often a history of some minor dental procedure or a blow to the face from which the onset of the pain is dated.

The pain is remarkably similar in site and quality from patient to patient and would be consistent with irritation of the second division (and sometimes third division) of the trigeminal nerve or its central connections. In the one patient of mine on whom an autopsy was performed (case history below) no pathological change was demonstrated other than the degeneration resulting from the surgical section of the second and third divisions of the trigeminal nerve. The condition is often associated with depression and the use of antidepressants provides partial relief in most patients. Electroconvulsive therapy has been reported as helping some patients. Others, like the patient whose history is recounted below, prove resistant to all forms of treatment including psychotherapy.

CASE REPORT

A patient with atypical facial pain

A man aged 53 years had suffered a single major epileptic seizure 20 years previously. Shortly after this the left upper gum started to ache and he was treated by washing out the left maxillary sinus and removing the nasal septum. Pain persisted since then, starting in the left upper gum near the midline and radiating upwards to the left nostril and the left cheek under the eye. It was barely noticeable in the early morning and became progressively worse during the day. A left carotid arteriogram and CSF examination in another hospital were found to be normal. A radical antrostomy did not provide relief. The left infra-orbital nerve was blocked with alcohol, and finally sectioned, without any benefit. The left cheek, nostril and upper lip felt numb since then but pain remained in the anaesthetic areas.

He had been subject to typical right-sided migraine headaches which had recurred every three months throughout his life. He said that he was a tense, worrying man who had felt depressed ever since his fit 10 years ago. He was treated with amitriptyline, 25 mg, three times daily and after 2 weeks said that the pain was reduced in severity and that he felt much brighter and could face life again. After 4 months' treatment, the pain was still present but he felt that he could now live with it satisfactorily. He had found that deliberately relaxing his jaw reduced his facial pain.

Over a period of 5 years his pain gradually returned to its former intensity. It was not benefited by intracranial section of the second and third divisions of the trigeminal nerve, by increasing the dose of amitriptyline to 150 mg daily or by mono-amine oxidase inhibitors. The sphenopalatine ganglion was blocked with cocaine and the stellate ganglion was injected with Xylocaine, producing a Horner's syndrome, without any change in the facial pain. Dr T. Torda infiltrated the upper cervical posterior roots, resulting in analgesia from the limits of the trigeminal distribution down to the fourth cervical segment without improvement. On another occasion Dr Torda induced an epidural block of posterior roots which extended from the fourth cervical segment down to the second thoracic segment but the pain persisted at the height of analgesia. Electroconvulsive therapy administered to the right hemisphere on 8 occasions over a period of 3 weeks did not help. A modified leucotomy diminished his awareness of the pain but it continued nevertheless. He died suddenly at the age of 53 from a pneumothorax caused by rupture of an emphysematous bulla.

At autopsy, the ventral surface of the brainstem was examined carefully to ensure that there was no compression of the trigeminal nerve by an aberrant artery. No abnormality was seen here or at the root entry zone in the pons apart from atrophy of the root resulting from previous surgery. A detailed histological examination was made of the pons, descending spinal tract and nucleus of the trigeminal nerve and thalamus by Dr A. Tait-Smith without any changes being found other than those attributable to surgery.

REFERRED PAIN

Eyes

Imbalance of the extra-ocular muscles (heterophoria), especially convergence weakness, or refractive errors, particularly uncorrected presbyopia, may set up 'eyestrain' headache, which is a form of tension headache following visual effort. This condition is much overdiagnosed and it is uncommon for headache to be cured simply by the correction of a visual disturbance. There are some odd ocular pains which do not seem to be of any significance, known as ophthalmodynia (Behrens, 1976). These are jabbing pains in one eyeball which may be repetitive, without obvious cause. Angle-closure glaucoma may cause pain to be felt deeply in the eye and to radiate over the forehead in the distribution of the first division of the trigeminal nerve. There may not be mistiness of vision, coloured haloes seen around lights or circumcorneal injection to draw attention to the eye. Radiation of pain from eye to forehead should arouse suspicion of glaucoma in the middle-aged or elderly patient and lead to a full ophthalmological examination including measurement of the intra-ocular tension.

Pain in or behind the eye is a common feature of retrobulbar neuritis and may precede impairment of vision by a few hours or even days. The pain radiates to the frontal region of the same side. Sight becomes blurred and may be lost completely in the affected eye. The most common visual field defect is a central scotoma since the central part of the optic nerve containing fibres from the macula is most often affected by the demyelinating process. It is probable that retrobulbar neuritis is always caused by primary demyelination of the optic nerve, and more than half the patients who suffer an attack subsequently develop signs of demyelination elsewhere in the nervous system. The exact percentage of patients who progress to typical multiple sclerosis varies greatly from series to series depending upon the criteria of diagnosis and the length of follow-up.

During the acute attack, the eyeball is often tender to pressure and aches on eye movement. The optic fundi are usually normal on ophthalmoscopic examination unless the area of demyelination underlies the nerve head, when swelling of the optic disc is observed. This inflammatory oedema, termed papillitis, is said to give a reddish appearance to the disc as well as the characteristic appearance of papilloedema. Distinction between the two conditions does not present any difficulty because vision is seriously impaired or lost in papillitis, whereas there is usually no more than slight blurring of vision on head movement with papilloedema, even when the disc is grossly swollen.

Both pain and visual disturbance of retrobulbar neuritis usually respond rapidly to the use of adrenocorticotrophic hormone (ACTH). A controlled trial of ACTH, 40 units daily, given for 30 days demonstrated that all 25 patients given the active substance were relieved of pain within 48 hours, some within a few hours (Rawson, Liversedge and Goldfarb, 1966). The control group of 25 patients continued to have pain for up to 2 weeks. Vision improved more rapidly in the treated group. At the end of 30 days, only 2 patients in the treated group were unable to read small print, compared with 12 of the untreated patients. There is evidence that demyelination responds better to ACTH than to adrenal corticosteroids, and it is possible that some substance other than cortisol, released from the adrenal cortex by ACTH, is responsible for the beneficial results. One patient of mine provided convincing evidence of the efficacy of ACTH in that pain diminished and vision returned within 24 hours of starting treatment with ACTH on three occasions. The first course of injections was ceased after about 1 week because the condition appeared to have subsided but pain and blindness returned 1 day afterwards. A second course of 2 weeks was equally effective but recurrence followed as soon as treatment was stopped. The third course was continued for 6 weeks, after which the patient remained symptom-free.

Ear, nose and throat

Vasomotor rhinitis is said to give rise to a midfrontal headache. The author is rather sceptical of this statement since vasomotor rhinitis is a common disorder and affects many patients and colleagues without causing headache. It does, of course, predispose to sinusitis, which causes headache in the stage of active inflammation or when the ostium of a particular sinus is obstructed.

The diagnosis of sinusitis rarely presents any difficulty when the pain and tenderness are localized to the affected frontal or maxillary sinus or sinuses and percussion over the area increased the pain. Inflammation of the ethmoid or sphenoidal sinuses gives rise to a boring pain felt deeply in the midline behind the nose (*Figure 6.3*). The pain of sinusitis is made worse by bending the head forwards. If the ostium to the infected sinus is patent, blowing the nose or sneezing usually evokes a throb of pain. If the ostium is obstructed, the patient may awaken with a 'vacuum' headache caused by absorption of air from the blocked sinus.

One or both nostrils are usually blocked and the maintenance of a clear airway by decongestants will lead to discharge of mucopurulent

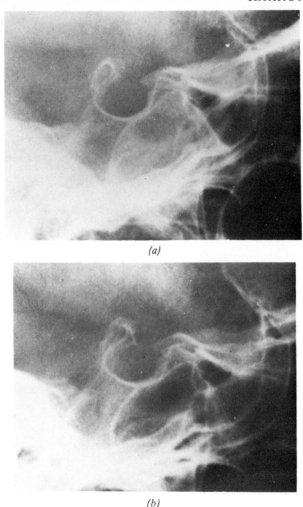

(a)

(b)

Figure 6.3. Sphenoidal sinusitis (a) before and (b) after treatment

material from the sinuses with subsequent relief of pain in most instances. The use of vasoconstrictor nose drops or nasal spray, such as neosynephrine 0.25 per cent every 2 to 3 hours, instilled first with the head postured backwards over the end of a bed, and then, after some minutes, with the head upright, will clear the airway in most patients. When the airway is clear, steam inhalation, followed by the application of radiant heat to the affected area, helps to clear the ostia. If symptoms of systemic disturbance appear, antibiotics may be required but the first requirement is to ensure that sinuses are draining freely. If this cannot be accomplished by the simple measures outlined, the advice of an ear, nose and throat surgeon should be obtained. Sinusitis is often taken lightly but may be treacherous if it persists, and lead to collections of pus in the extradural or subdural spaces, to cerebral abscess or to spread of infection through the bloodstream.

CASE REPORT

The following reports a patient with frontal sinusitis leading to extradural empyema, cerebral abscess and pyaemia.

A boy aged 16 years complained of right supra-orbital pain for 10 days before he was referred to the hospital because of increasing severity of headache and vomiting over the past few days. Apart

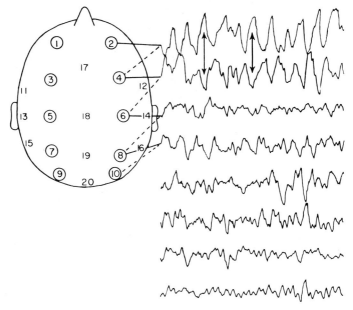

Figure 6.4 Electroencephalogram in cerebral abscess. The sketch on the left represents the head seen from above with the standard electrode placements and the origin of the tracings from the right hemisphere are indicated. High voltage slow waves are seen to arise in the right frontal region, with phase reversal (shown by arrows) demonstrating their origin from the right precentral electrode

from slight stiffness of the neck, no abnormality was found on admission to hospital. CSF pressure was found to be 140 mm and the fluid contained 250 cells/mm^3, half of which were polymorphonuclear, and a protein content of 90 mg/100 ml. He was considered to have a viral meningitis until a left-sided epileptic seizure 1 week after admission prompted a neurological consultation. On examination, the abdominal reflexes were found to be diminished on the left side and the left plantar response was less definitely flexor than the right. Radiographs demonstrated uniform opacity of the right frontal sinus and electroencephalograpic findings were typical of right frontal abscess with high voltage 2 Hz waves focal at the right precentral electrode (*Figure 6.4*). After this was confirmed by

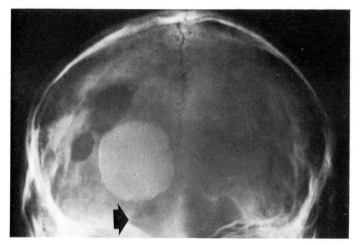

Figure 6.5. Intracerebral abscess arising from right frontal sinusitis (same patient as in Figure 6.4). The right frontal sinus (arrowed) is less radiolucent than the left. The abscess cavity is demonstrated by the injection of radio-opaque material after drainage through the burr holes which may be seen above and lateral to it. (Case history in text)

carotid arteriography, an extradural collection of pus was evacuated, followed by an operation on the frontal sinus, aspiration of an abscess in the right frontal lobe and finally aspiration of a purulent arthritis of a knee joint. The radiographic appearance of the right frontal sinus with the abscess cavity behind it is illustrated in *Figure 6.5*. The lad eventually made a complete recovery. The offending organism was staphylococcus aureus.

A mucocele may develop in one frontal sinus if the ostium of the sinus is obstructed and can slowly expand, eroding bone until it projects into the orbit, causing proptosis.

The cranial nerves are invaded by nasopharyngeal carcinoma more often than by any other malignant growth in the head and neck because of the proximity of the nasopharynx to the foramina of the middle fossa. The condition is rare in communities of European origin but is common in China and South-East Asia. The trigeminal nerve or its branches are involved in about half the cases, so that pain may be referred to the head. The sixth cranial nerve is also vulnerable and is destroyed in about 70 per cent of patients. In addition the ninth, tenth and eleventh cranial nerves may be invaded, causing hoarseness and dysphagia. Other symptoms include nasal obstruction, bloody nasal discharge and enlargement of cervical lymph nodes. About 40 per cent of patients present with headache.

CASE REPORT

The following is the case report of a patient whose headache was a diagnostic problem for 4 years before the diagnosis of naso-pharyngeal carcinoma became apparent.

A man aged 44 years was investigated in November, 1973, for constant pain in the right temple for the previous 4 years. The pain had since spread to the right eye and radiated to the occiput. It was not made worse by coughing, sneezing or head movement, and was partially relieved by oral administration of ergotamine tartrate.

Physical examination showed a partial right sixth nerve palsy and hypaesthesia most marked over the first division of the trigeminal nerve (Gradenigo's syndrome). This is usually caused by pathological changes at the apex of the petrous temporal bone; however, relevant investigations, including tomography, were reported to give normal results at this time. A biopsy of the superficial temporal artery also appeared normal.

The pain continued to get worse and in May, 1974, he complained of increasing numbness over the right side of his face and tongue. Radiographs taken at this time showed erosion of the base of the skull around the foramen ovale. Repeated tomography demonstrated destruction of the apex of the petrous temporal bone and floor of the middle fossa on the right side, indicating infiltration by carci-noma. The sphenoid sinus was opaque and the pituitary fossa was largely destroyed (*Figure 6.6*). Biopsy of the sphenoid sinus showed that this was an adenoid cystic carcinoma. Radiotherapy produced relief of pain within a few days, although his hearing loss and double vision had not been relieved. He remained well for twelve months after the course of radiotherapy but his pain recurred, necessitating thermocoagulation of the Gasserian ganglion.

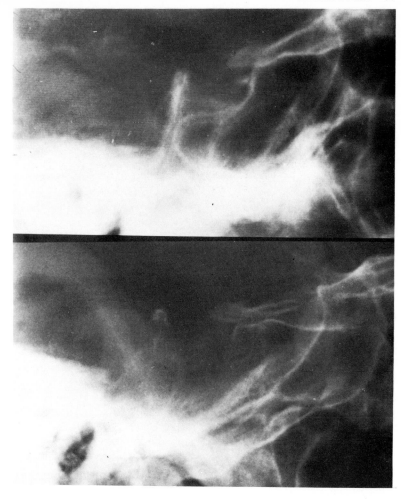

Figure 6.6. Radiographs of the pituitary fossa and the sphenoid sinus taken at an interval of 6 months showing erosion by nasopharyngeal carcinoma

Hippocrates warned that an association of headache with acute pain in the ear is to be dreaded 'for there is danger that the man may become delirious and die' (Adams, 1948). Otitis media may cause thrombosis of the lateral sinus and 'otitic hydrocephalus' (*see Figure 8.9*). Intracranial abscesses from middle ear disease are uncommon nowadays, but may be found in the temporal lobe or cerebellum and present with signs of raised intracranial pressure, focal neurological disturbance or meningeal irritation.

Teeth

Dental caries or apical root infection can cause a neuralgic pain in the second or third divisions of the trigeminal nerve, with a constant aching component and superadded jabbing pains. The pain is made worse by hot or cold fluids in the mouth. Pains in the lower jaw are almost always of dental origin and warrant careful radiographs of the teeth as apical root infections may be missed in a routine examination. Pains in the upper jaw are commonly of dental origin but can readily be produced by maxillary sinusitis.

A common way for dental disturbance to refer pain to the upper part of the head is through dysfunction of one temporomandibular joint. If the bite is unbalanced by premature contact of one or more teeth or by loss of molar teeth on one side, or if the bite is fixed so that the normal lateral or shearing movement of mastication is impossible, the patient adopts the most convenient chewing position, which commonly throws an abnormal strain on one temporomandibular joint. This may lead to pain which is felt in front of or behind the ear on the appropriate side with radiation to the temple, over the face, and down the neck on that side, often associated with a blocked sensation in that ear (Costen's syndrome) (Costen, 1934). The condition is made worse by the patient becoming a chronic 'jaw clencher' if he was not one already, so that tension symptoms are set up in the temporal and other scalp muscles. Ill-fitting dentures or any other source of discomfort in biting or chewing may evoke the same symptoms. In long-standing cases crepitus may be heard or felt over the affected temporomandibular joint.

The management depends upon careful adjustment of the bite by a dental surgeon, but advice to the patient concerning relaxation of the temporal and masseter muscles is also helpful. The problem is discussed further under the heading of Tension Headache (*see* page 114).

Neck

John Hilton (1950) made the following remarks in the fourth of a series of 18 lectures given on 'Rest and Pain' between 1860 and 1862.

Suppose a person to complain of pain upon the scalp, is it not very essential to know whether that pain is expressed by the fifth nerve or by the great or small occipital? Thus pain in the anterior and lateral part of the head, which are supplied by the fifth nerve, would suggest that the cause must be somewhere in the area of the distribution of the other portions of the fifth nerve. So if the pain be expressed behind, the cause must assuredly be connected with the great or small occipital nerve, and in all probability depends on disease of the spine between the first and second cervical vertebrae.

John Hilton (1805–1878)

Degeneration of the upper cervical disc spaces or deformity of the first two or three cervical vertebrae can cause compression of the appropriate posterior roots which refer pain to the occipital region.

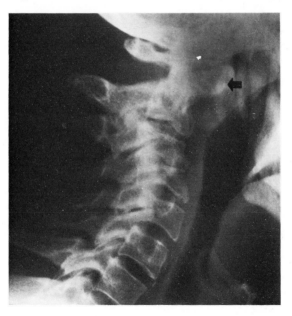

Figure 6.7. Deformity of the upper cervical spine in rheumatoid arthritis. The odontoid process (arrowed) is angulated forwards. The patient presented with occipital headache and signs of spinal cord compression

Pain is also experienced in the neck and, if the lower cervical spine is also affected, the shoulder girdle as well. The first and second vertebrae are commonly involved in advanced rheumatoid arthritis with angulation of the odontoid process and subluxation of the joints (*Figure 6.7*).

In addition to pain in the head and neck, spinal cord compression may be an indication for operative fixation of the upper cervical spine.

The contribution of changes in the lower cervical spine to generalized headache is more controversial. Stimulation of the upper cervical nerve roots may refer pain to the trigeminal distribution, but there is

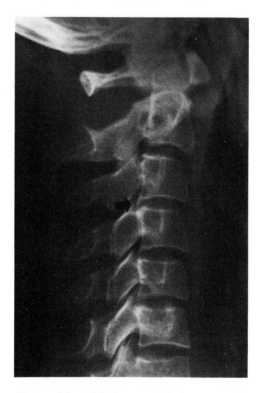

Figure 6.8. Mild degenerative changes in the cervical spine associated with headache referred to the eye. Disc spaces between the third and fourth, and fifth and sixth cervical vertebrae are slightly narrowed with posterior projection of osteophytes at the upper level (arrowed). Case history in text

no known means of referral of pain to the head from the lower cervical spine. One sees many patients with cervical spondylosis complaining of pain in the neck and shoulders, with paraesthesiae in the hands, who do not have headache. When headache is a symptom of such patients, its quality and associations are usually those of muscle-contraction (tension) headache, which may be initiated by concern over their neck condition or may be independent of it. It has been postulated that cervical spondylosis may damage the periarterial nerve plexus of the vertebral artery by osteophytes impinging on it, and hence set up diffuse headache, but this concept remains unproven. The occasional dramatic relief of headache by cervical manipulation must be balanced against those patients whose headache is unimproved and whose neck pain may be made worse by manipulative procedures. There are a few whose radiological signs of spondylosis are limited to the lower cervical spine but whose headache appears to be brought on or aggravated by neck movement and who are relieved by cervical traction.

CASE REPORT

The following presents a case of cervical spondylosis with referral of pain to the head and face.

A medical colleague aged 42 years had been subject to recurrent attacks of pain in the right shoulder since he was a student. After some years pain was experienced in the neck as well as the shoulder during these attacks and he noticed crepitus in the neck. At the age of 33 years he developed right sciatic pain with numbness of the sole, and a degenerated lumbosacral disc was removed by laminectomy. His neck and shoulder pain continued to recur several times a year. At the age of 41 years he noticed pain above, behind and below the right eye after playing golf. He attributed this to twisting his neck in fixing the golf ball with his left eye. The pain then became daily and was referred from the eye to the temple and ear on the right side. The pain was made worse by neck movement or by the vibration and jolting of car or air travel. When the pain became severe he had to hold his neck to the left, so as to extend the right side of the neck, to obtain relief. No abnormality was found on examination apart from stiffness and crepitus in the neck. Electroencephalography was within normal limits. Radiographs of the skull and sinuses were normal but those of the cervical spine disclosed degenerative changes at the disc space between the third and fourth cervical vertebrae (*Figure 6.8*). A right carotid arteriogram was done in view of the distribution of the pain and was normal. The headache eased gradually during a course of cervical traction. It has not recurred since although he has had further episodes of neck pain.

The contribution of the cervical spine to headache is discussed further in Chapter 14 (page 231).

REFERENCES

Adams, F. (1948). *The Genuine Works of Hippocrates*, p.54, London: Sydenham Society

Atkinson, R.A. and Appenzeller, O. (1975). Headache in small vessel disease of the brain: a study of patients with systemic lupus erythematosus. *Headache* 15, 198

Behrens, M.B. (1976). Headaches and head pains associated with diseases of the eye. *Res. Clin. Stud. Headache. (Basel:Karger)*. 4, 18

Chawla J.C. and Falconer, M.A. (1967). Glossopharyngeal and vagal neuralgia. *Br. med. J.* 2, 529

Costen, J.B. (1934). A syndrome of ear and sinus symptoms dependent upon disturbed function of the temporomandibular joint. *Ann. Otol. Rhinol. Lar.* 43, 1

Denny-Brown, D. and Yanagisawa, N. (1973). The function of the descending root of the fifth nerve. *Brain* 96, 783

Elliott, F.A. (1964). Treatment of herpes zoster with high doses of prednisone. *Lancet* 2, 610

Gillanders, L.A., Strachan, R.W. and Blair, D.W. (1969). Temporal arteriography A new technique for the investigation of giant-cell arteritis and polymyalgia rheumatica. *Ann. rheum. Dis.* 28, 267

Hilton, J. (1950). *Rest and Pain*, p. 77. Ed. by E.W. Walls and E.E. Philipp. London:Bell

Hunder, G.G. and Allen, G.L. (1974) The relationship between polymyalgia rheumatica and temporal arteritis. *J. Geriat.* (Feb), 35

Jannetta, P.J. (1973). Observations of the etiology of trigeminal neuralgia in 100 consecutive operative cases. Definitive microsurgical treatment by relief of compression-distortion of the trigeminal nerve at the brain stem. Paper delivered at Neurosurgical Congress, Tokyo.

Nathan, P.W. (1976). The gate-control theory of pain. A critical review. *Brain* 99, 123

Paulley, J. W. and Hughes, J.P. (1960). Giant-cell arteritis, or arteritis of the aged. *Br. med J.* 2, 1562

Raskin, N.H. (1976). Biologic correlates of migraine. In *Current Reports in Neurology*, p. 8. Rahway, Merck & Co.

Raskin, N.H. and Prusiner, S. (1977). Carotidynia. *Neurology* 27, 43

Rawson, M.D., Liversedge, L.A. and Goldfarb, G. (1966). Treatment of acute retrobulbar neuritis with corticotrophin. *Lancet* 2, 1044

Roseman, D.M. (1968), Carotidynia. In *Handbook of Neurology*. Vol. 5, Ed. P.J. Vinken and G.W. Bruyn, p. 375. Amsterdam:North Holland

Selby, G. (1975). Diseases of the fifth cranial nerve. In *Peripheral Neuropathy* Ed. P.J. Dyck, P.K. Thomas and E.H. Lambert, pp 533–569, Philadelphia: W.B. Saunders Co.

Shanbrom, E. (1961). Treatment of herpetic pain and postherpetic neuralgia with intravenous procaine. *J. Am. Med. Ass.* 176, 1041

Silberberg, D.H., and Laties, A.M. (1973). Increased intracranial pressure in disseminated lupus erythematosus. *Archs. Neurol.* 29, 88

Sweet, W.H. and Wepsic, J.G. (1974). Controlled thermocoagulation of trigeminal ganglion and rootlets for differential destruction of pain fibres. Part 1: Trigeminal neuralgia. *J. Neurosurg.* 40, 143

Toussaint, D. (1968). Raeder's syndrome. In *Handbook of Neurology*. Vol. 5. Ed. P.J. Vinken and G.W. Bruyn. Amsterdam: North Holland, 333

Wadman, B. and Werner, I. (1972). Observations on temporal arteritis. *Acta med. scand.* **192**, 377

Watkins, S.M. and Espir, M. (1969). Migraine and multiple sclerosis. *J. Neurol. Neurosurg. Psychiat.* **32**, 35

Seven

Simple Intracranial Vasodilatation

Headaches resulting from dilatation of intracranial vessels are characteristically throbbing in nature and made worse by jarring of the head or any sudden movement.

Intracranial vascular headache may be caused by head injury (post-concussional headache), circulating toxins in acute infectious febrile diseases and by pyrogenic agents such as typhoid vaccine. Hypoglycaemia may produce a vascular headache in some people who miss a regular meal-time or in those with carbohydrate intolerance in which case headache appears several hours after meals. Hypoxia and hypocapnia cause headache by increasing cerebral blood flow. Some medications such as indomethacin may cause a daily dull headache.

Headaches following epileptic seizures

Increased cerebral blood flow is probably responsible for the headache which follows a major (tonic-clonic) epileptic seizure. Plum, Posner and Troy (1968) have analysed the effects on the monkey cerebral circulation of the direct metabolic changes resulting from the seizure discharge itself and the indirect effects from alterations in respiration and muscle metabolism. Although the animals were anaesthetized, paralyzed and adequately ventilated with oxygen, cerebral blood flow increased during an induced seizure to a mean of 264 per cent over the resting level. This was caused by increased carbon dioxide production and loss of autoregulation of the cerebral blood vessels so that flow increased passively with the neurogenic elevation of blood pressure

70

accompanying a seizure. In spite of an increase in cerebral metabolism of 60 per cent, venous oxygen tension actually rose and there was no demonstrable cerebral acidosis. Similar findings in man have been reported by the same group of workers. In a spontaneous epileptic seizure, hypoxia from respiratory arrest is an added factor.

Acute mountain sickness

Headache is the most frequent and severe symptom of acute mountain sickness (King and Robinson, 1972). Of 30 young men subjected for 30 hours to simulated altitudes of 14 to 15 000 feet in a hypobaric chamber, 28 developed headache. This was usually bilateral but localized to one side in 25 per cent. The headache was relieved by compression of the superficial temporal arteries more completely than by the Valsalva manoeuvre, suggesting that the extracranial arteries were of more importance for the production of headache than intra-cranial vasodilatation. The cause of the headache was not necessarily hypoxia since similar headaches resembling migraine have been reported after exposure to a hyperbaric chamber. Other factors such as fluid and electrolyte changes may play a part. Spironolactone, an aldosterone antagonist, has recently been reported as preventing the headache of mountain sickness if taken prophylactically.

Histamine headache

Any agent which dilates the extracranial or intracranial arteries is likely to produce headache. Pickering and Hess (1933) found that the intravenous infusion of histamine caused flushing of the face followed by a generalized throbbing headache. Wolff (1963) and his colleagues showed that headache came on after the scalp arteries had returned to their normal calibre whereas CSF pulsation was still increased by 250 per cent while histamine headache was in progress. Increasing intra-cranial pressure to 1000 mm CSF relieved histamine headache immediately, confirming the idea that it was caused by dilatation of intracranial vessels rather than scalp arteries.

Nitrites and nitrates: 'hot dog headache'

When the inhalation of amyl nitrite was used for the treatment of angina pectoris it often caused a sudden bilateral throbbing headache as a complication of its vasodilator action. Glyceryl trinitrate may have the same effect in patients who are not usually subject to headache and is a reliable precipitating agent of cluster headache during a bout.

An uncommon but interesting variation on this theme is a headache that afflicts some unfortunate people after eating cured-meat foods. Nitrites are added to salt to give a uniform red appearance to cured meat. The concentration of nitrite in the meat when cooked is only 50 to 130 parts per million but this is sufficient to cause headache in some susceptible individuals after eating 'hot dogs', bacon, ham or salami. Henderson and Raskin (1972) described such a patient who developed headache on most occasions after ingesting 10 mg of sodium nitrite but not after a placebo of sodium barcarbonate.

Monosodium glutamate: 'the Chinese restaurant syndrome'

Headache has been reported as part of the Chinese restaurant syndrome (Schaumburg *et al.*, 1969) – a symptom complex of pressure and tightness in the face, burning over the trunk, neck and shoulders and a pressing pain in the chest which may follow 20 to 25 minutes after eating a Chinese meal. The headache, a pressure or throbbing over the temples and a band-like sensation around the forehead, has been attributed to monosodium glutamate (MSG) which is used abundantly in Chinese cooking. About 3 g of MSG, contained in 200 ml of wonton ('short') soup, may provoke headache in those sensitive to it.

Alcohol

Ethyl alcohol is of course a vasodilator agent and may trigger migraine or cluster headache in this way. The cause of 'hangover headache' which happens the day after excessive alcohol intake is still uncertain. The average rate at which a normal-sized adult metabolizes alcohol is about 10 ml/h (Ritchie, 1970). It is first oxidized to acetaldehyde by alcohol dehydrogenase, and acetaldehyde is then converted to acetyl-coenzyme A which is oxidized or used in the synthesis of cholesterol and fatty acids. Disulfiram, administered to discourage the intake of alcohol, increases the blood acetaldehyde concentration 5 to 10 times and produces the 'aldehyde syndrome'. The face becomes flushed and a throbbing headache may develop, associated with nausea, vomiting and giddiness, followed by hypotension and pallor. Whether the headache of a hangover can be attributed solely to acetaldehyde or other break-down products of alcohol remains unknown.

Marihuana

Dryness of the mouth, paraesthesiae, a sensation of warmth and suffusion of the conjunctivae are common after the ingestion of 60 mg of *cannabis sativa*. Five out of 10 subjects studied by Ames (1958) complained of mild frontal headache, presumably related to vasodilata-tion. I have had patients tell me that tension headache is relieved by smoking marihuana so that its relaxing and vasodilator properties may combine to help this form of headache just as alcohol does.

Rebound headache

Unlike vasodilators, vasoconstrictor agents do not in themselves induce headache, but a rebound dilatation may follow the constriction induced by nicotine as the result of excessive tobacco smoking or the vasocon-strictor effect of caffeine contained in tea, coffee, or commercial analgesic preparations. As the effect of the last dose wears off, a dull headache may become apparent which is relieved by repeating the dose, one of the factors in habituation. The injudicious use of ergotamine tartrate in the treatment of vascular headaches that recur frequently can lead to a similar problem which is discussed later in the section on migraine.

Pressor reactions in patients taking MAO inhibitors

There have been many reports of patients under treatment with mono-amine oxidase (MAO) inhibitors who have experienced sudden severe headache, often occipital in site, following the administration of amphetamines or drinking red wine or eating cheeses with a high tyra-mine content. The headaches are associated with a rapid increase in blood pressure and are relieved by the alpha-noradrenergic blocking agent, phentolamine. Some cases of subarachnoid haemorrhage have occurred at the height of the pressor reaction. Foods which contain large amounts of mono-amines and sympathomimetic drugs must therefore be avoided by patients taking MAO inhibitors. We issue a sheet of instructions to all patients prescribed MAO inhibitors stating that they must not take cheese, meat extracts such as Marmite, red wines, broad beans, chicken livers (pâté) or pickled herrings (rich in tyramine). They are prohibited from having any injections or tablets other than those prescribed specifically for headache such as ergotamine, aspirin or codeine. The use of a nasal decongestant spray containing sympathomimetic agents is to be avoided.

Phaeochromocytoma

A rare but interesting cause of acute pressor reactions is phaeochromocytoma. Thomas, Rooke and Kvale (1966) reviewed the clinical histories of 100 patients with proven phaeochromocytoma seen at The Mayo Clinic in the preceding 20 years. Episodic headache was a feature of the attacks in 80 per cent. It was usually of rapid onset, bilateral, severe, throbbing and was associated with nausea in about half the cases. The headache lasted less than one hour in 70 per cent and was accompanied by other symptoms of catecholamine release in 90 per cent.

Recently, Dr Hinterberger and I (Lance and Hinterberger, 1976) analysed the case histories of 27 patients in whom Dr Hinterberger had studied the content of adrenaline (A) and noradrenaline (NA) in blood, urine and the tumour after it had been removed. We were unable to find any distinctive syndrome for tumours producing predominantly one of these amines. Sustained hypertension was more common in the NA-secreting group while pallor and tremor were more common when adrenaline was produced by the tumour as well. Other symptoms such as palpitations, sweating and anxiety were present in both groups. Headaches, which appeared to be related to a rapid increase in blood pressure, were a symptom in 20 of the 27 patients and had the same characteristics as those previously described by Thomas, Rooke and Kvale (1966). Blood pressure recorded during a headache ranged from 200/100 mm Hg to 300/160 mm Hg. However blood pressures as high as 260/160 mm Hg had been recorded in some patients who were not subject to headache. Two patients with bladder phaeochromocytoma experienced severe headache 15 to 20 seconds after micturition, that lasted 1 to 3 minutes. Others described the headache as lasting for a few seconds or minutes only at the onset of their paroxysmal symptoms but mostly the headache persisted for 5 minutes to 2 hours, subsiding gradually with the other symptoms of the attack. Nausea and vomiting accompanied the headache in 7 patients and 2 complained of blurred vision. Six patients had collapsed, lost consciousness or developed focal neurological signs during the episodes. Attacks were provoked by exertion, straining, emotional upsets, worry or excitement. High levels of circulating catecholamines cause uptake and storage in other adrenergic tissue including the adrenal medulla, from which they are released on nervous stimulation. This accounts for paroxysmal symptoms being triggered by anxiety and excitement as well as by compression of the tumour.

The diagnosis depends on clinical suspicion being aroused when the history is first taken and is confirmed by finding increased excretion of catecholamines in three 24-hour specimens of urine, or elevated blood levels during an attack. Care must be taken that the patient has not taken any sympathomimetic drugs preceding the urine collection, nasal decongestant sprays being the most consistent offender. Blood sugar is usually elevated at the time of the attack, a useful distinction from hypoglycaemic attacks which may simulate phaeochromocytoma because of the secondary release of adrenaline in hypoglycaemia. The tumour is localized by intravenous pyelography and aortic angiography if it is present in the characteristic suprarenal site. It must be borne in mind that phaeochromocytomas may arise at any point along the line of development of the sympathetic chain, extending downwards from the neck to the pelvis and scrotum.

Headaches related to sexual activity

Headaches developing during sexual excitement are considered immediately after acute pressor reactions because the severe headache which may occur at the moment of orgasm has similar characteristics to that described in phaeochromocytoma. The association of headache with 'immoderate venery' was first pointed out by Hippocrates (Adams, 1939). Sexual intercourse has been known to precipitate subarachnoid haemorrhage but it is important to recognize that the occurrence of headache at this time is not necessarily indicative of serious intracranial disorder.

There are three kinds of headache associated with sexual activity. The first is a dull headache, commonly bilateral and occipital in site, that comes on as sexual excitement mounts. It is probably related to excessive contraction of head and neck muscles since it can be prevented or relieved by deliberate relaxation of these muscle groups. The second type of headache, more severe and explosive in onset, appears immediately before or at the moment of orgasm, presumably caused by the increase in blood pressure at this time. A third type, which I have not encountered, was described by Paulson and Klawans (1974) in 3 of their 14 patients with headaches arising during coitus.

This form of headache was worse on standing up and thus resembled the low pressure headache following lumbar puncture, leading the authors to postulate that the arachnoid membrane may have been torn during the physical stress of coitus.

This condition affects men more than women and may occur at any time during the years of sexual activity. It is capricious in that it may develop on several occasions in succession then not trouble the patient again although there is no obvious change in sexual technique. In my own experience of 25 patients, 19 were male and 6 female, aged from 18 to 58 years. Four patients experienced headache with masturbation, three of whom also complained of similar headaches during sexual intercourse. The headaches of the remaining patients were confined to sexual intercourse. Those patients who desisted from sexual activity when headache was first noticed found that it subsided within a period of 5 minutes to 2 hours. Those who proceeded to orgasm reported that a severe headache persisted for 3 minutes to 4 hours and a milder headache lingered for 1 to 48 hours afterwards (Lance, 1976).

The headaches were more likely to occur when intercourse was attempted for a second time after a brief interval. One young man complained of headaches at orgasm while he was on holiday for a month, indulging in sexual intercourse two or three times daily. When the holiday was over and the frequency of intercourse declined to once daily he remained free of headache. Carotid and vertebral angiography was performed in some of the first patients I saw with this syndrome and was completely normal. As familiarity with the syndrome increased, I have reserved this investigation for those patients in whom there was suspicion of an underlying lesion. One of my patients, a young man aged 25 years, had symptoms of a mild brainstem infarction with perioral numbness, paraesthesiae in the arms and double vision. Two other older patients had experienced symptoms of vascular insufficiency unrelated to intercourse. With these exceptions, there has been no detrimental effect from the headaches and follow-up for periods of up to 9 years has not disclosed any underlying structural lesion. Thus there appears to be a 'benign sex headache' analogous to benign cough headache and benign exertional headache. Benign sex headache is not a form of exertional headache since it may come on when the subject is not exerting himself or herself and is playing a completely passive role. Blood pressure has been recorded as high as 214/135 mm Hg in normotensive subjects at the time of orgasm (Littler, Honour and Sleight, 1974) so it is not remarkable that headache may develop at this time as an acute pressor response. Because of the occasional occurrence of vascular complications any patient experiencing a headache during sexual intercourse would be well advised to desist on that particular occasion.

Exertional and cough headache

The quotation from Hippocrates (Adams, 1939) alluded to above reads in full 'one should be able to recognize those who have headaches from gymnastic exercises, or running, or walking, or hunting, or any other unseasonable labour, or from immoderate venery.' Sharp pain in the head on coughing, sneezing, straining, laughing or stooping has long been regarded as a symptom of organic intracranial disease, commonly associated with obstruction of the CSF pathways. Sir Charles Symonds (1956) presented the case histories of 6 patients in whom cough head-ache was a symptom of a space-occupying lesion in the posterior fossa or of basilar impression from Paget's disease. He then described 21 patients with the same symptom in whom no intracranial disease became apparent. Cough headache disappeared in 9 patients and improved spontaneously in another 6 patients. Two patients died of heart disease and 4 were lost to follow-up. Symonds concluded that there was a syndrome of *benign cough headache* which he attributed to the stretching of a pain-sensitive structure in the posterior fossa, possibly the result of an adhesive arachnoiditis. Of Symond's 21 patients, 18 were males and ages ranged from 37 to 77 years, with an average age of 55. Williams (1976) recorded CSF pressures from the cisterna magna and lumbar region during coughing. He found that there was a phase in which lumbar pressure exceeded cisternal pressure followed by a phase in which the pressure gradient was reversed. He postulated that cough headache may be caused by a valve-like blockage at the foramen magnum which interferes with the downward or rebound pulsation.

Rooke (1968) considers that cough headache is a variety of exertional headache and recorded his experience with 103 patients who experienced transient headaches on running, bending, coughing, sneezing, lifting or straining at stool, in whom no intracranial disease could be detected and who were followed for 3 or more years. During the follow-up period, reinvestigation discovered structural lesions in 10 patients, such as Arnold—Chiari malformation, platybasia, subdural haematoma, and cerebral or cerebellar tumour. Of the remaining 93, 30 were free of headache within 5 years and 73 were improved or free of headache after 10 years. This type of headache was found in men more often than women in the ratio 4:1. The aetiology is unknown but Rooke observes that this form of headache may appear for the first time after a respiratory infection with cough and that some patients reported an abrupt recovery after the extraction of abscessed teeth, which had also been noted by Symonds.

I would prefer to maintain the separation between *'benign cough headache'* and *'benign exertional headache'* (which is more common in a younger age group). Exercise may precipitate typical severe migraine headache in some patients, and the usual headache following exercise has the pulsatile quality of vascular headache resembling a mild migrainous episode. One patient of mine, a young athlete, who had developed such a headache at the end of each training session, could prevent it by taking ergotamine tartrate, 1 mg, orally before training began each day. Others have found that methysergide, 1–2 mg, taken the night or morning before the planned exercise was equally effective.

Hypertension

There is no doubt that a sudden rise of systemic blood pressure can cause headache. Acute pressor reactions caused by phaeochromo-cytoma, MAO inhibitors and sexual intercourse are described above. Such headaches are usually bilateral, affecting the occipital or frontal areas, and may involve the whole head. They are commonly severe, 'bursting' or throbbing in quality, and associated with other symptoms of catecholamine release, such as tremor or palpitations. The increase in blood pressure in acute nephritis or malignant hypertension may also take place rapidly enough to cause headache.

Whether the insidious onset of hypertension can be responsible for headache is less certain. The typical headache ascribed to hypertension by various writers over the past 60 years is bilateral, usually occipital in site, present on waking and easing as the patient gets up and about. Wolff (1963) pointed out that the headache associated with hypertension may respond to rest and relaxation without any material change in blood pressure. Symptoms of anxiety are common in hypertensive patients once they know that their blood pressure is elevated and muscle contraction headache may be a manifestation of this anxiety. There have been remarkably few controlled studies to determine the effect of blood pressure alone on the incidence of headache.

A community survey (Waters, 1971) involving 414 people, of whom 36 had a systolic pressure greater than 195 mm Hg and 13 had a diastolic pressure higher than 115 mm Hg, disclosed no difference in the prevalence of headache between the small hypertensive group and the control subjects. On the other hand, Bulpitt, Dollery and Carne (1976) found that 31 per cent of untreated hypertensive patients complained of headaches on waking compared with 15 per cent of normal subjects and treated hypertensive patients, a statistically significant difference. The headache improved more often in those patients whose blood pressure dropped substantially on treatment.

Badran, Weir and McGuiness (1970) studied a group of 100 patients with a blood pressure of 150/95 mm Hg or more and 100 matched normotensive controls. Headache was a symptom in 50 hypertensive patients and 39 controls. Headache was significantly more common in hypertensive patients only when the diastolic pressure was 140 mm Hg or more. Eight of 12 patients with papilloedema had headache. Of the 11 patients in the grossly hypertensive group, only 2 experienced occipital headache, the remainder being bitemporal or diffuse. Oddly enough, occipital headache was more common in the control group, affecting 20 of the 39 patients. The headache of gross hypertension did indeed occur in the mornings, eased after several hours and improved in those whose blood pressure responded to treatment. Bauer (1976), in a retrospective survey of 400 patients, could not find any significant correlation between the height of blood pressure and the incidence of headache. A follow-up extending to 15 years showed that there was no difference in mortality between those with headache and those without.

It may be tentatively concluded that hypertension by itself is not a common cause of headache but that there is an association between these disorders which may lead to improvement in headache with control of hypertension.

What of the relationship between hypertension and migraine? Walker (1959) found that hypertension was significantly more common in migrainous patients over the age of 50 years. Leviton, Malvea and Graham (1974) compared the frequency of hypertension and vascular disease in migrainous and non-migrainous parents of patients with migraine. 'High blood pressure' was significantly more common in the migrainous parents (whether men or women) in a ratio of 1.7 : 1 ($p < 0.05$). The incidence of heart attacks under the age of 70 years was almost three times higher in the migrainous parents ($p < 0.05$), irrespective of whether or not they were hypertensive. Curiously, the tendency to stroke was not increased.

Headache during haemodialysis

Bana, Yap and Graham (1972) reported that 70 per cent of 44 patients had experienced headache during haemodialysis. Six patients described typical muscle-contraction headaches and 11 of 12 migrainous patients had their usual headache precipitated by dialysis. The authors described a new entity 'dialysis headache' which started a few hours after the procedure as a mild bifrontal ache and later became throbbing, sometimes accompanied by nausea and vomiting. The severity of the headache was related to hypertension, excessive sodium intake and emotional upsets. The occurrence of headache at a predictable time gives an opportunity to study various humoral factors which could be responsible. Arterial renin levels are lower in these patients subject to headache and lower still at the time of headache (Graham, personal communication). Dialysis headache appears to be of vascular origin and is responsive to small doses of ergotamine.

Cerebral vascular disease

Headache is a prominent symptom in approximately 25 per cent of patients with transient ischaemic attacks. Grindal and Toole (1974) analysed the nature of the headache of 56 patients in whom the site of origin of the ischaemic episodes had been determined. Of 33 patients with carotid insufficiency, the headache was ipsilateral to the diseased carotid in 9, contralateral in 2 and bilateral in the remainder, commonly affecting the frontal region. Ipsilateral frontal or orbital pain followed visual disturbance in 4 out of 5 cases of amaurosis fugax. Headache in vertebrobasilar insufficiency was more consistently associated with the ischaemic attacks and affected the occiput or neck in 15 out of 23 cases.

Fisher (1968) reported that 31 per cent of patients with internal artery occlusion have some pain or discomfort, most often a unilateral frontal ache. In contrast to the authors quoted above, he did not obtain a history of headache in any of his 58 patients with transient monocular blindness. Thrombosis or embolism of the middle cerebral artery was accompanied by headache in about 20 per cent of cases, in the frontotemporal area on the affected side. Headache was more common in posterior cerebral artery occlusion, affecting 71 per cent of patients, usually lateralized to the side of the thrombosis. In lateral medullary infarction, pain from ischaemia of central trigeminal pathways had to be distinguished from the headache caused by vascular occlusion which was usually occipital in site. The fact that the headaches associated with vascular occlusion are commonly unilateral suggest that some local factor is involved but no satisfactory explanation has been postulated. There is no evidence that collateral circulation is any greater in patients with headache than in those without headache.

The headache of cerebral embolism is probably caused by vascular distension. *Figure 7.1* shows a mycotic aneurysm in a patient with subacute bacterial endocarditis who presented with left-sided headaches associated with transient aphasia and right hemiparesis. The diagnosis was complicated by a past history of migraine. Subacute bacterial endo-carditis was confirmed by blood cultures but in spite of a satisfactory response to antibiotics, the patient developed intensely severe headache and died rapidly two weeks after the onset of her illness. At autopsy, the vegetations on the mitral valve were found to be healing satisfactorily. The left hemisphere was expanded by a large intra-cerebral haematoma. Immediate operation is now advocated for mycotic aneurysm.

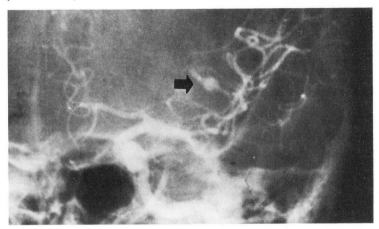

Figure 7.1. Mycotic aneurysm situated peripherally on a branch of the middle cerebral artery. The patient presented with transient left-sided headaches, aphasia and right hemiparesis as the result of cerebral embolism from subacute bacterial endocarditis

There have been a few reports of an intense vascular headache, localized to the frontotemporal area of the affected side, following carotid endarterectomy (Pearce, 1976). The headache comes on after a latent period of 36 to 72 hours and recurs intermittently for 1 to 6 months. It seems unlikely that the headache could be caused simply by the restoration of normal cerebral perfusion pressure and it may be related to some disturbance in the carotid arterial wall. West, Davies and Kelly (1976) reported a distinctive headache syndrome in 8 patients with narrowing or occlusion of one internal carotid artery, shown to be caused by a dissecting aneurysm of the arterial wall in 1 operated case. The pain was unilateral and was associated with a Horner's syndrome on the same side and often with contralateral neurological symptoms or signs in half the patients. The pain involved the head, neck or face and had a burning or throbbing quality. It subsided over a period of two months.

These syndromes have been placed in a chapter on 'simple cranial vasodilatation' for convenience because pain receptors within the arterial wall appear to play an important part in their production.

REFERENCES

Adams, F. (1939). The genuine works of Hippocrates. p. 94. Baltimore: Williams and Wilkins

Ames, F. (1958). A clinical and metabolic study of acute intoxication with *cannabis sativa* and its role in the model psychoses. *J. ment. Sci* **104**, 972

Badran, R.H.Al., Weir, R.J. and McGuiness, J.B. (1970). Hypertension and headache. *Scott. Med. J.* **15**, 48

Bana, D.S. Yap, A.U. and Graham, J.R. (1972). Headache during hemodialysis. *Headache* **12**, 1

Bauer, G.E. (1976). Hypertension and headache. *Aust. N.Z. Jl Med.* **6**. 492

Bulpitt, C.J., Dollery, C.T. and Carne, S. (1976). Change in symptoms of hypertensive patients after referral to hospital clinic. *Br. Heart. J.* **38**, 121

Fisher, C.M. (1968). Headache in cerebrovascular disease. In *Handbook of Clinical Neurology*, Vol. 5, p. 124. Amsterdam: North Holland

Grindal, A.B. and Toole, J.F. (1974). Headache and transient ischaemic attacks. *Stroke* **5**, 603

Henderson, W.R. and Raskin, N.H. (1972). Hot-dog headache: individual susceptibility to nitrite. *Lancet* **2**, 1162

King, A.B. and Robinson, S.M. (1972). Vascular headaches of acute mountain sickness. *Aerospace Med.* (August) 849

Lance, J.W. (1976). Headaches related to sexual activity. *J. Neurol. Neurosurg. Psychiat.* **39**, 1226

Lance, J.W. and Hinterberger, H. (1976). Symptoms of phaeochromocytoma, with particular reference to headache, correlated with catecholamine production. *Archs Neurol.* **33**, 281

Leviton, A., Malvea, B. and Graham, J.R. (1974). Vascular diseases, mortality, and migraine in the parents of migraine patients. *Neurology* **24**, 669

Littler, W.A., Honour, A.J. and Sleight, P. (1974). Direct arterial pressure, heart rate and electrocardiogram during human coitus. *J. Reprod. Fert.* **40**, 321

Paulson, G.W. and Klawans, H.L. (1974). Benign orgasmic cephalgia. *Headache* **13**, 181

Pearce, J. (1976). Headache after carotid endarterectomy. *Br. med. J.* **3**, 85

Pickering, G.W. and Hess, W. (1933). Observations on the mechanism of headache produced by histamine. *Clin. Sci.* **1**, 77

Plum, F., Posner, J.B. and Troy, B. (1968). Cerebral metabolic and circulatory responses to induced convulsions in animals. *Archs Neurol.* **18**, 1

Ritchie, J.M. (1970) The aliphatic alcohols. In *The Pharmacological Basis of Therapeutics.* 4th edition, Ed. L.S. Goodman, and A. Gilman, p. 135. London: Collier Macmillan

Rooke, E.D. (1968). Benign exertional headache. *Med. Clins N. Am.* **52**, 801

Schaumburg, H.H., Byck, R., Gerstl, R. and Mashman, J.H. (1969). Monosodium L-glutamate. Its pharmacology and role in the Chinese restaurant syndrome. *Science, N.Y.* **163**, 826

Symonds, C.P. (1956). Cough headache, *Brain* **79**, 557

Thomas, J.E., Rooke, E.D. and Kvale, W.F. (1966). The neurologist's experience with pheochromocytoma: a review of 100 cases. *J. Am. med. Ass.* **197**, 754

Walker, C.H. (1959). Migraine and its relationship to hypertension. *Br. med. J.* **2**, 1430

Waters, W.E. (1971). Headache and blood pressure in the community. *Br. med. J.* **1**, 142

West, T.E.T., Davies, R.J. and Kelly, R.E. (1976). Horner's syndrome and headache due to carotid artery disease. *Br. med. J.* **1**, 818

Williams, B. (1976). Cerebrospinal fluid pressure changes in response to coughing. *Brain* **99**, 331

Wolff, H.G. (1963). *Headache and Other Head Pain.* London and New York: Oxford University Press

Eight

Intracranial Causes of Headache

And he said to his father, my head, my head. And he said to a lad, carry him to his mother. And when he had taken him, and brought him to his mother, he sat on her knees till noon, and then died.

(2 Kings **IV**, 19–20)

Walton (1956) suggests that this may be an early recorded case of subarachnoid haemorrhage. If so, the unusual sequel is worth noting. The prophet Elisha was summoned and as he was approaching he was met with the news that 'there was neither voice, nor hearing . . . the child is not awaked'. Elisha 'went up and lay upon the child, and put his mouth upon his mouth . . . and the flesh of the child waxed warm . . . . The child sneezed seven times, and the child opened his eyes'.

The sudden onset of headache, followed by loss of consciousness with recovery after resuscitation, makes a dramatic early description of headache of intracranial origin whether the cause was subarachnoid haemorrhage, as Walton suggests, or another intracranial disorder such as encephalitis.

MENINGEAL IRRITATION

The presence of blood in the subarachnoid space causes an inflammatory response in the meninges, probably because of the release of chemical agents. Heparinized whole blood does not produce pain when applied to a blister base, unless it has been retained in a syringe for several minutes. In these circumstances platelets break down and release serotonin, and the plasma kinin-forming system is activated. The pain of injury or inflammation, as well as the pain provoked by extravascular

84

blood, appears to be caused by the concerted action of substances which are contained in whole blood and are formed from inactive plasma precursors. Serotonin and kinins are probably the most important in this respect.

The chemical excitation of nerve endings in the meninges produces a reflex spasm of the neck extensors and sometimes of the lumbar muscles, which is analogous to the contraction of the abdominal wall resulting from peritoneal inflammation, and known as muscle 'guarding'. Muscle spasm consequent upon meningeal irritation gives rise to the physical signs of neck rigidity and Kernig's sign.

Subarachnoid haemorrhage

Bleeding into the subarachnoid space may take place after head injury, or secondary to an intracerebral haemorrhage or 'spontaneously' in patients with cerebral aneurysm or angioma. Less commonly, bleeding may be the result of blood dyscrasias, haemorrhage from cerebral tumour, or some form of arteritis. The ratio of aneurysm to angioma as a cause of subarachnoid haemorrhage varies in different Western series from 5:1 to 25:1. The pattern is quite different in Asia, where angioma is more common. The headache of subarachnoid haemorrhage follows exertion in about one-third of patients. It usually starts suddenly and dramatically, 'like a blow on the head'. There may be a poorly localized sensation of something giving way inside the head, followed by unilateral headache which rapidly becomes generalized and spreads to the back of the head and neck, accompanied by photophobia. The patient may lose consciousness, with or without an epileptic seizure. The neck is usually rigid, and focal neurological signs are found if the aneurysm has compressed cranial nerves in enlarging or has bled into the brain substance (*Figures 8.1 and 8.2*). Pain in the back and legs may follow a subarachnoid haemorrhage after some hours or days, because of blood irritating the lumbosacral nerve roots. Haemorrhages may be seen in the fundi, spreading out from the optic discs, in some 7 per cent of patients, and papilloedema is found in 13 per cent (Walton, 1956). Fever, albuminuria, glycosuria, hypertension and electrocardiographic changes may be present in the acute phase.

The diagnosis is made clinically and confirmed by lumbar puncture, when uniformly blood-stained fluid is withdrawn. After 4 to 12 hours, xanthochromia of the cerebrospinal fluid becomes apparent and it disappears from 12 to 40 days after the haemorrhage. A lymphocytic cellular reaction and increase in CSF protein to 70–130 mg/100 ml usually follows subarachnoid haemorrhage (Walton, 1956).

When the patient is conscious, it is best to arrange for transfer as

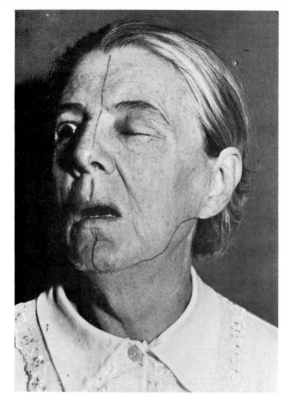

Figure 8.1. Loss of sensibility over the left half of the face with a complete left ptosis (third cranial nerve palsy). The onset was sudden with intense pain behind the left eye

soon as practicable to a neurological centre for cerebral angiography and surgical treatment should a suitable vascular malformation be demonstrated. If no aneurysm or angioma can be found, the patient is confined to bed for 4 to 6 weeks, and resumes normal activities gradually.

The relationship of aneurysm and angioma to migraine

Of 220 patients with arteriovenous malformations or angiomas diagnosed by carotid angiography at the National Hospital for Nervous

Diseases, London, 12 (5 per cent) were found to have a history of migraine (Blend and Bull, 1967). In Walton's series of 312 cases of subarachnoid haemorrhage, 16 (5 per cent) gave a definite history of migraine. Six of his patients lost their migraine attacks after the episode of haemorrhage. Davis (1967) found that 6 per cent of 431 patients presenting with subarachnoid haemorrhage had a migrainous history.

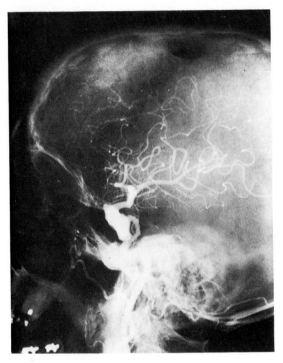

Figure 8.2. Left carotid angiogram of the patient in Figure 8.1., showing a large aneurysm arising from the carotid siphon in a suitable position to compress the third cranial nerve and all three divisions of the trigeminal nerve

The incidence of 5 to 6 per cent in these series is not very different from that of the general population. In contrast, Wolff (1963) found that 7 out of 46 patients with subarachnoid haemorrhage had suffered from migraine and another 12 had periodic recurrent headaches. However, the side of the aneurysm did not always relate to the side of the headache, and Wolff considered that the headache was independent of the presence or absence of aneurysm. Other studies have reported a

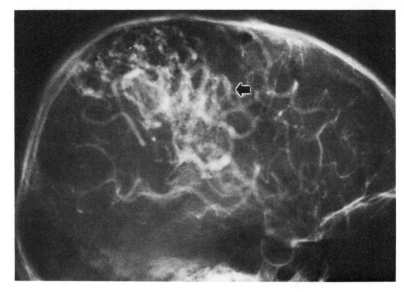

Figure 8.3. A large arteriovenous malformation demonstrated by carotid angiography in a young woman who suffered from classic migraine and repeated subarachnoid haemorrhages. (Case history in text)

migraine history of 15 per cent of 110 patients (Patterson and McKissock, 1956) and 31 per cent of 48 patients (Waltimo, Hokkanen and Pirskanen, 1975). The last figure was derived after careful questioning of all patients about their previous headache pattern. It remains uncertain from published statistics whether the association between migraine and intracranial vascular malformations is more than could be expected by chance. Certainly carotid arteriography is not indicated solely because migraine attacks habitually affect the same side of the head. If the patient also has a loud intracranial bruit, or is subject to focal fits affecting the opposite side of the body, or has had a subarachnoid haemorrhage, then the likelihood of a positive result from carotid angiography is greatly increased. Some patients with cerebral angiomas have repeated small subarachnoid haemorrhages which are confused with migraine attacks or are thought to be episodes of 'encephalitis'.

CASE REPORT

The following is a case of cerebral angioma presenting as migraine with repeated subarachnoid haemorrhage.

A trained nurse aged 24 years had suffered from migraine head-ache since the age of 8 years. The attacks recurred about once a month and were always preceded by a sensation of 'pins and needles' spreading over the left side of the body. This sensation lasted for 10 to 30 minutes and was followed by a throbbing right-sided headache and nausea. The early administration of oral ergotamine tartrate aborted the majority of attacks. At the age of 13 years she had a particularly severe episode with neck stiffness and drowsiness which was thought to be a viral meningo-encephalitis. When aged 18 years she experienced a severe pain in the back of the neck followed by vomiting and neck stiffness. This pain eased but later she developed a severe right frontal headache with left-sided paraesthesiae which persisted for 2 hours. On examination her neck was rigid and a bruit was heard over both orbits, louder on the right side. A lumbar puncture disclosed uniformly blood-stained fluid and carotid angio-graphy demonstrated an extensive intracerebral angioma (*Figure 8.3*). Since then she has been maintained on methysergide 1 mg three times daily and has been subject to three or four typical migraine headaches each year. She has continued to have episodes of subarachnoid haemorrhage at intervals of 3 to 24 months without any permanent neurological deficit.

Meningitis and encephalitis

The headache of intracranial inflammation may rarely present so acutely as to resemble subarachnoid haemorrhage, but more com-monly the onset is gradual over hours or days. The pain is bilateral, extends down the neck, is associated with photophobia, and is made worse by head movement. The patient commonly has a fever and neck stiffness on examination.

The diagnosis is made by clinical assessment and lumbar puncture. The CSF contains an excess of cells, mostly neutrophils in pyogenic infections and in the acute phase of some cases of viral encephalitis. A purely lymphocytic pleocytosis usually indicates a viral infection but may be found in some cases of tuberculous or cryptococcal meningitis. A low CSF glucose value (in the absence of hypoglycaemia) means that the infecting organism is metabolizing glucose and indicates a pyogenic, tuberculous or torular infection. An exception to this rule is the unusual condition of meningitis carcinomatosa in which the meninges are infiltrated and ensheathed with malignant cells which multiply so rapidly that the CSF glucose level drops. The reticuloses and secondary melanoma may present in this way and the author has seen several cases of primary sarcoma of the meninges with a meningitic onset and multiple nerve root involvement.

Postpneumo-encephalographic reaction

The introduction of air or oxygen into the subarachnoid space for diagnostic purposes (pneumo-encephalography, air encephalography, air study) leads to a sterile inflammatory reaction which occasionally simulates meningo-encephalitis in its severity. Samples of CSF taken during or after the air study often show a lymphocytic pleocytosis. In the more severe cases, the patient complains of photophobia and neck stiffness and may vomit so that the physician thinks of the possibility of meningitis induced by contamination at the time of lumbar puncture. The author has never seen this happen, whereas sterile reactions following pneumo-encephalography are not uncommon. The inflammatory response is superimposed on the natural tendency to headache after lumbar puncture, caused by the lowered CSF pressure. The reaction is generally less in patients with large cerebral ventricles resulting from cerebral atrophy and is always greater when air passes over the surface of the cerebral hemispheres in the subarachnoid space. Some patients are free of headache the day after an air study but others continue to have headache for as long as 7 to 14 days after the procedure. The introduction of methylprednisolone acetate, 40 mg, into the CSF at the conclusion of the air study reduces the frequency of unpleasant reactions. Apart from this the only therapeutic measures are to administer analgesics as required, to keep patients lying flat in bed and encourage them to drink a lot of fluid until the headache subsides. A similar reaction may occur after myelography and is handled the same way.

TRACTION ON, OR DISPLACEMENT OF, INTRACRANIAL VESSELS

Space-occupying lesions

Unless a tumour or other space-taking lesion occupies a strategic position along the line of the drainage pathways of the cerebral ventricles, it is able to reach a considerable size before causing headache. Since the intracranial vessels have to be pushed aside before pain is registered, infiltrating tumours such as the gliomas may extend throughout one hemisphere without causing headache, because the position of large vessels may remain undisturbed until the last stages of the disease. Tumours which compress the brain from outside, such as meningiomas, are likely to cause fits, focal cerebral symptoms, progressive impairment of intellectual function or other neurological deficit before they produce headache. Headache is an initial symptom in about one-third of patients with intracranial tumours but is present in 80 per cent of patients by the time the tumour is diagnosed (Rushworth, 1960).

Subdural haematoma, on the other hand, advances on a wide front so that a large surface area of brain is forced inwards and downwards. It almost invariably presents with headache, usually accompanied by drowsiness, and must be suspected in any patient of any age in whom these symptoms have progressed steadily over some days or weeks, even in the absence of a history of head injury. When the condition is well advanced, the patient usually develops a hemiparesis on the side opposite the subdural haematoma. Occasionally the hemiparesis is on the same side as the lesion because the midbrain has been displaced by the expanding mass so that the opposite cerebral penduncle impinges on the tentorium. The author has seen in some patients a bilateral spastic weakness of the limbs. The third nerve, which crosses from mid-brain to the cavernous sinus, is stretched as the enlarging mass forces part of the temporal lobe down through the tentorial opening on that side. Signs of a third nerve palsy (ptosis, enlarged pupil, failure of the eye to adduct or elevate fully) are therefore indications for immediate action because midbrain compression and irreversible damage are not far away.

CASE REPORT

The following is a case of subdural haematoma with quadriparesis resulting from a trivial injury.

A woman aged 48 years was holidaying in Noumea when she became aware of a right frontal headache which was worse on sudden movement of the head. The pain became worse over 12 days so that she returned to Sydney. She was drowsy but able to give a clear history, and could not recollect any head injury in the past 2 years. On examination of the fundi, the optic cups were indistinct and there was no venous pulsation. There was an incomplete third nerve palsy on the right. Flexor groups were weak in both lower limbs, with increased deep reflexes and extensor plantar responses. Immediate carotid angiography disclosed a large right subdural haematoma which was removed later that evening. When she had recovered her normal mental acuity she recalled that 6 weeks previously she had stood up suddenly in the kitchen, banging her head on an open cupboard door, which made her 'see stars' for a moment.

Extradural haematoma usually results from tearing of the middle meningeal artery at the site of a fracture and presents a more acute

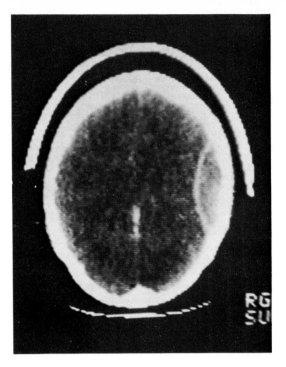

Figure 8.4. Extradural haematoma demonstrated by computerized tomography

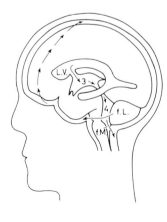

Figure 8.5. Diagram of the circulation of the cerebrospinal fluid from its origin in the choroid plexus, through the ventricular system to its absorption from the subarachnoid villi of the superior sagittal sinus, after its passage in the subarachnoid space over the cerebral hemispheres. Obstruction at any point of the conducting system may increase intracranial pressure and lead to hydrocephalus. L.V. = lateral ventricle. 3,4 = third and fourth ventricle, respectively. f.L. = foramen of Luschka. f.M. = foramen of Magendie

problem. Diagnosis is confirmed by computerized tomography or angiography (*Figure 8.4*).

Increased intracranial pressure

Any lesion which obstructs the flow of CSF from the lateral ventricles through the foramen of Monro, third ventricle, aqueduct, fourth ventricle and its exit foramina, or prevents the passage of CSF over the cortex to its absorption site (*Figure 8.5*), will cause a rapid increase in intracranial pressure so that headache becomes the main presenting symptom.

A tumour in the vicinity of the third ventricle may also interfere intermittently with the function of the midbrain reticular formation so that posture cannot be maintained and the patient thus suffers from 'drop attacks,' in which he or she slumps heavily to the ground.

CASE REPORT

The following is a case of colloid cyst of the third ventricle presenting with headache, myoclonus and drop attacks.

A bank officer aged 36 complained of bilateral headache for the past 6 years, which extended down the neck and usually recurred every day, although there had been breaks of up to one week without headache. The pain was brought on by standing suddenly and lasted from 1 hour to the whole day. It was associated with slight blurring of the periphery of both visual fields and often with the 'jim-jams'. The 'jim-jams' either occurred on their own for 5 to 10 minutes, usually around noon, or preceded a headache. They consisted of trembling and weakness of the arms and legs, which caused him to drop things, and at times his legs buckled so that he had to support himself with his arms. On one occasion he lost consciousness suddenly without warning. He had always been a worrier, had lost four children at birth or shortly afterwards from Rh incompatibility and thought that he was becoming depressed like his mother who had recently been treated by electroconvulsive therapy. Physical examination and an electroencephalogram were normal. He did not report again for 12 months, at which time he had been confused and drowsy for 2 weeks. He was found to have bilateral papilloedema, a left grasp reflex and extensor plantar responses. Carotid angiography and ventriculography revealed an internal hydrocephalus caused by tumour of the third ventricle. A colloid cyst was removed through the foramen of Monro. After 1 week of akinetic mutism the patient recovered well and returned to work after some months although his memory remained impaired.

Stenosis of the aqueduct leading from the third ventricle to the fourth may be a congenital malformation which does not produce any symptoms until some systemic infection causes proliferation of its ependymal lining which then blocks the canal and produces an acute internal hydrocephalus.

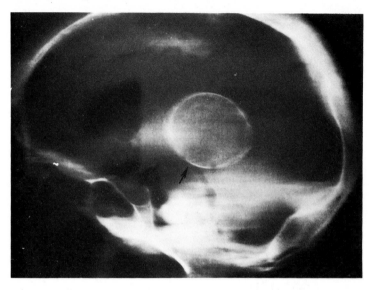

Figure 8.6. Calcified tumour obstructing the aqueduct

The aqueduct may also be obstructed by tumours in the vicinity of the midbrain (*Figure 8.6*).

Posterior fossa lesions

The aqueduct and fourth ventricle may be displaced or blocked by tumours of the posterior fossa. It is remarkable that tumours may grow to considerable size in the confined space of the posterior fossa without producing much in the way of symptoms or signs. The author has seen children and adults with large cystic astrocytomas and haemangioblastomas of the cerebellum whose only symptom apart from headache was unsteadiness of gait. There is no point in giving details here of the various types of posterior fossa tumours and the ways in which they may present. A unilateral nerve deafness warrants full investigation whether or not there are any other neurological symptoms because eighth nerve tumour should be diagnosed at an early stage, years before it is in a position to cause headache. Diplopia, facial paraesthesiae or pain, vertigo, ataxia, or any disturbance of speech or swallowing mechanisms obviously warrant investigation as soon as such symptoms appear.

A posterior fossa tumour may cause pain by direct compression of the fifth, seventh, ninth or tenth cranial nerves which may refer pain to the face, ear or throat. Pain is experienced in the neck because of irritation of the dura which is supplied by the upper three cervical nerve roots and reflex spasm of neck muscles may cause the head to be held to one side. Pain may also be referred to the eye and forehead by convergence of impulses from the upper cervical nerve roots upon neurones of the cervical cord which also serve the trigeminal pathways. Finally, a generalized headache may be caused by blockage of the flow of CSF with resulting increase in intracranial pressure. Some of these points are illustrated by the following protocol.

CASE REPORT

The following is a case of posterior fossa meningioma presenting with pain in the neck.

A woman aged 53 years noticed that her neck felt stiff when she looked up to hang clothes on a line, and that it ached when she was overtired. Since there was radiographic evidence of cervical disc degeneration, she was treated by cervical traction and manipulation which made the pain a little worse. One year later she began to be awakened from sleep at 2 to 3 a.m. about once a week by a bilateral headache which lasted for an hour. Neck pain persisted and, after another year had passed, occipital and frontal headaches were recurring daily. She then noticed a continuous dull ache in the left side of her face associated with a feeling of numbness involving the roof of her mouth on the left, which gradually crept over the cheek and the forehead. She felt nauseated and vomited without reason, which was attributed by the patient to nervous tension. The pain in her neck and back of the head became more severe and was particularly unpleasant after jolting or driving in a car. She noticed that she had to swallow twice to get food down, even after chewing it carefully, and she was a little unsteady on her feet at times.

On examination the optic fundi were normal. The left corneal reflex was depressed and 2-point discrimination was impaired on the left upper lip. Fine movements of the left arm and leg were a little clumsier than one would expect but there were no frank cerebellar signs. Carotid and vertebral angiography disclosed an internal hydrocephalus with a tumour circulation in the posterior fossa. On posturing the patient for posterior fossa craniotomy, the cardiac rhythm and respiration became irregular and remained so until the occipital bone was removed. A pressure cone of cerebellum was then seen to extend some 5 cm down the spinal canal to the third cervical vertebra. After removal of the posterior arch of the atlas and the spine and laminae of the second cervical vertebra, heart rate and respiration returned to normal. A large meningioma, approximately 4 cm in diameter, was found to be compressing the cerebellum and cranial nerves and extending through the tentorium. It was satisfactorily removed, and another operation two months later was required to remove its equally large supratentorial extension. The patient recovered well and slowly resumed her usual activities. She remains well 8 years after operation.

A haemorrhage into the cerebellum can rapidly prove fatal if not recognized and treated surgically, because it compresses respiratory and vasomotor centres in the brainstem. The condition may readily be confused with vertebrobasilar insufficiency or thombosis

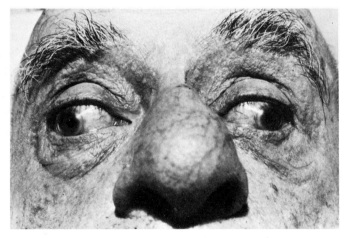

Figure 8.7. Deviation of the visual axes in an elderly patient with an acute intracerebellar haematoma, which was successfully removed. The patient recovered well but was left with severe ataxia of gait

because it is liable to occur in the middle-aged or elderly hypertensive patient and presents with sudden severe occipital headache, vertigo, ataxia and vomiting. Nystagmus or deviation of the visual axes may be found on examination (*Figure 8.7*), together with inco-ordination of upper and lower limbs and ataxia. The patient usually becomes stuporous or unconscious so that the diagnosis may have to be made on the history of the onset. Posterior fossa craniotomy is the only measure which will prevent the patients's death. Like intracerebellar haemorrhage, a subdural haematoma in the posterior fossa is uncommon, but it is worth mentioning because it is a remediable condition which must be thought of before it can be diagnosed.

Hydrocephalus may progress slowly from conditions in the region of the cisterna magna and foramen magnum. Tumours in this area, a congenital malformation known as the Dandy–Walker syndrome, and platybasia may be responsible for obstruction of the flow of CSF.

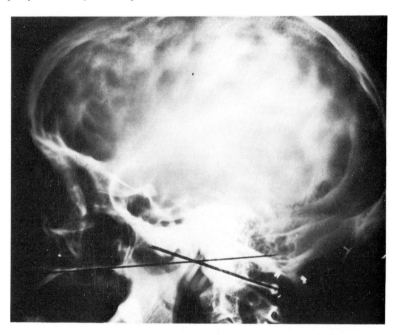

Figure 8.8. Radiological signs of long-standing hydrocephalus in a patient with congenital platybasia. The skull has a 'beaten-copper' appearance ('thumbing' of the vault), and the posterior clinoid processes are decalcified by pressure from the dilated third ventricle. The lines drawn through the body of the atlas and in the plane of the hard palate intersect at an angle of more than 13 degrees, one of the criteria for the diagnosis of platybasia

Platybasia is a flattening of the floor of the posterior fossa with rotation of the anterior parts of the atlas and axis upwards so that a line drawn through the body of the atlas forms an angle of more than 13 degrees with the line of the hard palate (Bull, Nixon and Pratt, 1955) (*Figure 8.8*). It may be a congenital anomaly, often associated with spina bifida, or may develop through softening of the base of the skull in Paget's disease, osteoporosis or osteomalacia.

Communicating hydrocephalus

The conditions so far considered produce an internal hydrocephalus with dilatation of the ventricular system on the central side of the block. Less commonly, the fluid may emerge freely from the fourth ventricle by the foramina of Magendie and Luschka but be impeded from ascending through the basal cisterns and subarachnoid space because of adhesive arachnoiditis. It has long been recognized that this may be a cause of hydrocephalus in tuberculous or other meningitis, but only recently it has been shown that the condition may develop quietly in the older patient, causing dementia. Progressive arachnoiditis may follow head injury or subarachnoid haemorrhage, or arise without obvious reason. The condition is suspected if pneumo-encephalography or CT scan demonstrates a large ventricular system, without widening of the cortical sulci which is pathognomonic of cerebral atrophy. The diagnosis is confirmed by brain scanning after the insertion of a radio-active isotope into the CSF to determine its rate of clearance from the ventricular system. Like other forms of hydrocephalus the condition may improve following insertion into the lateral ventricle of a catheter, which is then run under the skin of scalp and neck to be inserted through the jugular vein into the right antrium. The CSF thus drains into the venous circulation and a plastic valve prevents blood from passing into the CSF should the venous pressure become elevated.

Venous sinus thrombosis and otitic hydrocephalus

The lateral sinus may thrombose following infection of the middle ear and mastoid bone, causing cerebral oedema, termed 'otitic hydro-cephalus' (*Figure 8.9*). There is no internal hydrocephalus since the ventricles are normal or small in size. The patient, usually a child, develops headache and papilloedema after an ear infection. The sixth nerve may be paralyzed on the side of the lesion, or on both sides because of the nerves being stretched by the expanded brain. Radiographs commonly show opacity of the mastoid air cells. Treatment is directed to the infected ear and mastoid (which may include

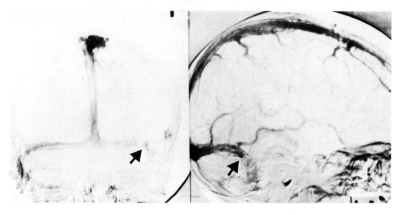

Figure 8.9. Lateral sinus thrombosed at apex of petrous temporal bone causing otitic hydrocephalus

mastoidectomy and removal of clot from the lateral sinus) and to reducing cerebral oedema.

CASE REPORT

The following is the report of a case of 'otitic hydrocephalus' with bilateral sixth nerve palsy.

A boy aged 4 years developed a typical attack of measles. Nine days after the disappearance of the rash he awoke during the night with pain in the right ear, and vomited. He was treated with tetracycline but complained of headache and noises in the head for the next 24 hours. He was admitted to hospital because of further vomiting and a slight increase in temperature. His fundi were normal, his right ear drum was reddened and there was slight neck stiffness. A lumbar puncture disclosed that his CSF was completely normal. He continued to have a mild fever and bilateral headache and developed a loose cough with occasional vomiting. Antibiotic treatment was altered to penicillin and then to ampicillin. One week after the onset of pain in the right ear, he was found to have a bilateral sixth nerve palsy and papilloedema. Radiographs of the skull showed opacity of the mastoid air cells on the right side. Ventriculography demonstrated that the lateral ventricles were smaller than normal. He recovered rapidly following ventricular drainage and mastoidectomy. Frusemide was used to reduce intracranial pressure after the ventricular drain was removed, and lumbar puncture confirmed the effectiveness of this treatment.

Raised venous pressure

Mediastinal obstruction and emphysema are said to increase venous pressure sufficiently to interfere with cerebral venous drainage and cause papilloedema. Hypoxia associated with these conditions probably increases the tendency to oedema of the brain and optic nerve.

Cerebral oedema from other causes

A sudden elevation of the blood pressure, as in malignant hypertension, may cause headache, presumably through the mechanism of cerebral oedema displacing pain-sensitive blood vessels, since the headache is relieved by the intravenous infusion of hypertonic solutions such as 50 per cent glucose but not when CSF pressure is reduced by lumbar puncture (Wolff, 1963). One hemisphere may swell following infarction, as a result of thrombosis of the internal carotid artery, or thrombosis or embolism of one of its main branches. Headache is commonly a symptom of cerebral infarction. Cerebral oedema may be sufficiently pronounced to cause papilloedema after internal carotid thrombosis, thus simulating an acute presentation of cerebral tumour.

Cerebral oedema used to be a major problem after craniotomy but is now controlled by the use of adrenal corticosteroids in high dosage, for example dexamethasone, 32–64 mg daily. Potent diuretics such as frusemide, 40–120 mg daily, are also valuable in the control of cerebral oedema. The oral administration of urea and glycerol and intravenous infusions of mannitol and glycerol have enjoyed popularity at various times.

Hypocalcaemia may produce cerebral oedema, papilloedema and fits. Prolonged dosage with corticosteroids has been reported as causing headache, vomiting, papilloedema, diplopia and drowsiness. Addison's disease may also be responsible for cerebral oedema and papilloedema (Jefferson, 1956).

CASE REPORT

The following is the report of a case of Addisonian crisis with meningeal irritation and papilloedema, simulating meningo-encephalitis.

A woman aged 32 years had her sixth child uneventfully but was unable to breast-feed her baby for more than a few days, which was unusual for her. About 1 month later she developed headache, rigors and vomiting, which cleared up without any treatment, although she continued to have slight bilateral headaches. Her husband noted that she was more irritable than usual and rather vague in her manner. Several weeks later she complained of a sore throat and awoke one night with severe headache, rigors and vomiting, and became drowsy. Her general practitioner gave her an intravenous injection of tetracycline and arranged for her transfer by ambulance. When admitted to the hospital, she was stuporous, restless and irritable, curling up to avoid the light. She was moderately pigmented on exposed areas with a prominent linea nigra and dark nipples, but there was no buccal pigmentation. Her colouring was thought to be consistent with being a country-dweller in a sunny climate, particularly as she had recently completed a pregnancy. Neck stiffness, Kernig's sign and early bilateral papilloedema were noted. Her blood pressure was 130/80 mmHg. On lumbar puncture, the flow of CSF was slow and the pressure could not be measured. The fluid contained 100 polymorphonuclear cells and 60 lymphocytes/mm^3, and a protein content of 80 mg/100 ml. Serum electrolytes were normal apart from sodium which was 130 mEq/litre. Radiographs of skull and chest and carotid arteriography were normal. She was thought to have a partly-treated bacterial meningitis or viral meningo-encephalitis, and penicillin, chloramphenicol and sulphadiazine were administered, although no organism was grown from CSF or blood cultures. Her temperature reached 39.5°C on several occasions and her blood pressure fell alarmingly to 80/50 mmHg. A repeated lumbar puncture showed that CSF pressure was 110 mm. The cellular and protein content was similar to that of the previous day and glucose content was 60 mg/100 ml. Corticosteroids were withheld because of the presumed infectious nature of her illness and she died that evening. Autopsy revealed that the brain was macroscopically and microscopically normal. There was a purulent pericarditis. The only adrenal tissue found was a sliver 2 mm thick on the right side which showed almost complete loss of adrenal cortex on histological examination.

Benign intracranial hypertension

This term is applied to a condition in which CSF pressure is raised without any demonstrable brain tumour, obstruction to the CSF pathways or venous sinus thrombosis. The insidious onset of generalized headache and sometimes nausea is associated with papilloedema. Paresis of one or both sixth cranial nerves develops in about 40 per cent of cases, presumably because the nerves are displaced and compressed by cerebral oedema. The condition is termed benign because life is not threatened but vision becomes permanently impaired in one-quarter of untreated cases because of postpapilloedema optic atrophy (Foley, 1955; Jefferson and Clark, 1976; Johnston and Paterson, 1974a).

Foley (1955) described two groups of patients, one in which the condition followed non-specific infections and mild head injuries and a larger group, mostly obese young women in whom there was no obvious cause. Benign intracranial hypertension has also been reported as a reaction to certain drugs such as tetracycline and nalidixic acid, as the result of excessive intake of vitamin A and as a sequel to the withdrawal of corticosteroid therapy.

The condition must be clearly distinguished from otitic hydrocephalus which it resembles closely. Benign intracranial hypertension appears to be caused by a reduction of CSF absorption since the production of CSF is normal while total CSF volume increases. Intracranial pressure builds up in waves followed by a sudden fall, suggesting that the increased pressure periodically forces fluid through the arachnoid villi. The various causative factors mentioned may all increase resistance to CSF flow across the villi (Johnston and Paterson, 1974b).

Confirmation of the diagnosis depends upon the demonstration of a normal ventricular system by CT scanning (or angiography followed by air encephalography if a CT scanner is not available). The condition is treated by salt restriction and diuretics, the efficacy of which can be checked by measuring the CSF pressure by lumbar puncture in the early stages of treatment, at which time CSF can be withdrawn to reduce the pressure if necessary. Papilloedema, which may be conveniently monitored by measuring the size of the blind spot on a Bjerrum screen, may resolve within 6 weeks. (Jefferson and Clark, 1976). About 80 per cent of cases return to normal within 3 months but 10 per cent may take 12 months or more. With adequate dehydration therapy it is rarely if ever necessary to perform operations such as bilateral subtemporal decompression or slitting the optic nerve sheath in order to preserve vision. The lesser procedure of inserting a shunt from the lateral ventricles to the right atrium via the internal jugular vein may be indicated if CSF pressure does not fall with diuretic therapy. Some 10 per cent of cases may recur. The obese female patient should lose weight but there is ample evidence that she may undergo pregnancies in the future without increasing her risk of recurrence.

Reduced intracranial pressure

The headache which often follows lumbar puncture is probably caused by continued leakage of CSF from the subarachnoid space after the procedure, which lowers intracranial pressure, withdrawing support for the brain, thus causing traction upon intracranial vessels. The frequency of such headaches may be reduced by using a fine-gauge needle, lying the patient on his front for 4 hours after lumbar puncture and maintaining bed-rest for 24 hours afterwards. Should a headache ensue, there is no treatment other than keeping the patient lying flat in bed, requesting him to drink as much fluid as possible and administering analgesics when required. A rare condition, known as spontaneous hypoliquorrhoea (Labadie, Antwerp and Bamford, 1976), may produce the same symptoms as the result of CSF leakage from an unknown source or from excessive absorption of CSF.

REFERENCES

Blend, R. and Bull, J.W.D. (1967). The radiological investigation of migraine. In *Background to Migraine,* p.1. Ed. by R. Smith. London: Heinemann

Bull, J.W.D., Nixon, W.L.B. and Pratt, R.T.C. (1955). The radiological criteria and familial occurrence of primary basilar impression. *Brain* 78, 229

Davis, E. (1967). Subarachoid haemorrhage. *Med. J. Aust.* 2, 12

Foley, J. (1955). Benign forms of intracranial hypertension – 'toxic' and 'otitic' hydrocephalus. *Brain* 78, 1

Jefferson, A. (1956). A clinical correlation between encephalopathy and papilloedema in Addison's disease *J. Neurol. Neurosurg. Psychiat.* 19, 21

Jefferson, A. and Clark, J. (1976). Treatment of benign intracranial hypertension by dehydrating agents with particular reference to the measurement of the blind spot area as a means of recording improvement. *J. Neurol. Neurosurg. Psychiat.* 39, 627

Johnston, I. and Paterson, A. (1974a). Benign intracranial hypertension. I. Diagnosis and prognosis. *Brain* 97, 289

Johnston, I. and Paterson, A. (1974b). Benign intracranial hypertension. II. CSF pressure and circulation. *Brain* 97, 301

Labadie, E.L., Antwerp, J. Van, and Bamford, C.R. (1976). Abnormal lumbar isotope cisternography in an unusual case of spontaneous hypoliquorrheic headache. *Neurology,* 26, 135

Paterson, J.H. and McKissock, W. (1956). A clinical survey of intracranial angiomas with special reference to their mode of progression and surgical treatment: a report of 110 cases. *Brain* 79, 233

Rushworth, R.G. (1960). Headache as a symptom of intracranial expanding lesions. *Bull. Post Grad. Comm. Med. Univ. Sydney* 16, 161

Waltimo, O., Hokkanen, E., Pirskanen, R. (1975). Intracranial arteriovenous malformations and headache. *Headache* 15, 133

Walton, J.N. (1956). *Subarachnoid Haemorrhage.* Edinburgh/London: Livingstone

Wolff, H.G. (1963). *Headache and Other Head Pain.* London and New York: Oxford University Press

Nine

Muscle-Contraction ('Tension') Headache

In peace there's nothing so becomes a man
As modest stillness and humility:
But when the blast of war blows in our ears,
Then imitate the action of the tiger;
Stiffen the sinews, summon up the blood,
Disguise fair nature with hard-favour'd rage;
Then lend the eye a terrible aspect;
. . . . let the brow o'erwhelm it . . . .
Now set the teeth and stretch the nostril wide . . . .

King Henry V, III, i

The staring eyes, furrowed brows and clenched teeth are appropriate enough in a man preparing for battle. A grimly set visage can be quite a handicap when it is the constant accompaniment of everyday life. When the sinews are stiffened in reaction to a crisis, physiological mechanisms 'summon up the blood' to supply the contracting muscles. When the muscles of a tense patient cannot stop contracting, the flow of blood through them may not be sufficient to prevent pain and herein may lie the cause of tension headache.

CLINICAL FEATURES

Incidence, age and sex distribution

Most people have probably been aware of a dull headache at some time of their lives after exposure to glare, flickering light, eyestrain, noise or a succession of harassing incidents. The number of persons who often experience such headaches must be considerable, judging from the sale of headache tablets and powders. The incidence of tension headaches which are frequent enough to warrant referral to a neurological clinic is almost as great as that of migraine. Over a period of 2½ years, 1 152 patients were referred to one out-patient clinic with the complaint of headache. Of these 612 suffered from migraine and 466 from tension headache (Lance, Curran and Anthony, 1965).

It is well known that migraine often begins in childhood but it is surprising to find that about 15 per cent of patients with tension headache also remember that their symptoms started before the age of 10 years (*Figure 9.1*). The condition may be intractable and persist throughout life. Many patients have suffered from headaches almost every day for 10, 20 or 30 years (*Figure 9.2*). As in the case of migraine, roughly 75 per cent of patients with chronic tension headache are women.

Family history

Some 18 per cent of patients with tension headache give a family history of migraine (Lance and Anthony, 1966), which is much the same as for the general population. However, a family background of some form of headache is found in the history of 40 per cent of tension headache patients (Friedman, Von Storch and Merritt, 1964).

Past health

There is no evidence that allergic disorders, childhood vomiting attacks or other disabilities are more common in patients complaining of tension headache than in the general community.

Site of headache

Muscle-contraction headache is bilateral in about 90 per cent of patients (Friedman, Von Storch and Merritt, 1964). It may be unilateral in patients who have imbalance of the bite. If a patient has a few back teeth missing on one side, or if the teeth cannot move freely from side to side, the bite is locked or distorted. The patient tends to

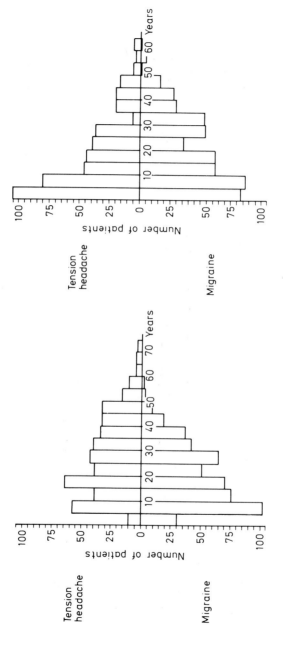

Figure 9.1. The age of onset of tension headache and migraine,
from Lance, Curran and Anthony (1965)

Figure 9.2. Duration of symptoms at the time of presenting
to a neurological clinic

(Reproduced by courtesy of the Editor of The Medical Journal of Australia)

chew on one side, throwing the strain onto one or other temporomandibular joint, so that the pain is felt in front of the ear and radiates over the temple.

Chronic jaw-clenchers commonly complain of pain over the contracting temporal and masseter muscles. The constant frowners have bifrontal headache and the 'stiff-necks' describe occipital pain. These sites may flow into one another so that the patient feels pain 'all over the head'.

Quality of headache

The pain is usually dull and persistent in tension headache, and undulates in intensity during the day. It is often described as a feeling of heaviness, pressure or tightness rather than pain and may extend like a band around the head. Some patients experience sudden jabs of pain on one side or at the back of the head superimposed on a general background of discomfort. About one-quarter of tension headache patients, whose headaches become severe and assume a pulsating quality at times, form a group intermediate between muscle-contraction headache and migraine which is called 'tension-vascular headache' (Lance and Curran, 1964). It is not uncommon for the headache to be throbbing on awakening but to settle down to its usual uniform character on starting the day's activities. About 10 per cent of patients with tension headache are also subject to frank migraine.

Time and mode of onset

In milder cases, the headache develops during or after recognizable stress. It may thus arise as a housewife gets her children off to school and her husband off to work; or while a driver battles with peak-hour traffic; or when the business executive is trying to juggle interviews and telephone conversations with the knowledge that he has not read the agenda for that meeting at 5 p.m. In more severe cases, the headache comes on in anticipation of some unpleasant situation, such as a distasteful interview. Contemplation of the day's tasks may be enough to start a headache while travelling to work by train. Immediately before the projected battle with Tweedledee, Tweedledum remarked 'I'm very brave generally, only today I happen to have a headache'.

In the most chronic form, the patient either awakens with the headache or notices it shortly after getting up and it remains throughout the day, without regard to the emotional content of the day's activities. Some 10 per cent of patients, not necessarily those who are depressed, may be woken up by tension-vascular headache between 1 a.m. and 4 a.m. in the manner of a migrainous patient.

Frequency and duration

Of 466 patients attending our neurological clinic for the treatment of tension headache, the headache recurred less than 10 times each month in 48 patients, from 10 to 30 times each month in 64 patients and was present every day in the remaining 354 patients (Lance and Curran, 1964). Friedman and his colleagues (Friedman, Von Storch and Merritt, 1964) found that 50 per cent of their patients experienced headaches every day. It is apparent that those patients attending clinics are those who are most severely affected and that figures from clinics do not necessarily reflect the pattern of tension headache as seen by the general practitioner. The spectrum of tension headache extends from headaches of 1 hour's duration recurring every few months to a perpetual unremitting ache present 'all day and every day'.

Associated phenomena

Muscle-contraction headache is not accompanied by any of the focal neurological symptoms which add a distinctive character to most attacks of migraine. There is often a constant mild photophobia, not severe enough to make the patient retreat to a darkened room but often sufficient to encourage the wearing of sunglasses on all but the gloomiest day. Other symptoms are those of an anxiety state. Slight nausea may be present in the early mornings, or when the headache is severe, but vomiting is rare. Giddiness or light headedness usually indicates a tendency to over-breathe in times of anxiety. Abdominal distension, excessive belching and passing of flatus are commonly the result of unnoticed air-swallowing. The patient often speaks of difficulty in concentrating and a lack of interest in work or hobbies. There may be more flagrant depressive symptoms which are attributed to the presence of headache. Pain under the left breast, pain in the back or coccygeal region, and indigestion are other psychosomatic symptoms commonly associated with tension headache. The patient may awaken with a bruised sensation inside the mouth lateral to the posterior upper molar tooth as the result of extreme mandibular movements during sleep (Every, 1960).

Underlying, precipitating, aggravating and relieving factors

It is deceptively easy to think of patients with tension headache as having an inadequate personality. This is certainly true of some patients who are ill-equipped by nature or education to cope with life's ramifications, but there are others who have considerable achievements to their credit. It may be that the meticulous energetic personality which has made a man prey to tension headache has also made him a leader in industry. A review by Martin, Rome and Swenson (1967) concludes: 'There does not seem to be a single psychologic determinant productive of muscle-contraction headaches. Multiple conflicts are usually evident in patients . . . poorly repressed hostility is often evident, but unresolved dependency needs and psychosexual conflicts are also frequently present . . . . . However, it seems that the psychophysiologic expression at somatization of anxiety in the form of increased skeletal-muscle tension is uniformly present in cases of muscle-contraction headache.'

In the author's own experience, approximately one-third of patients with tension headache have symptoms of depression (Lance and Curran, 1964). Most are conscious of the fact that they are never really relaxed and are rarely elated. Many patients with tension headache are 'born two drinks down on life'.

There may be obvious trigger factors for tension headache but in many patients the headache is not limited to times of emotional overload. The headache is usually made worse by any superadded anxiety, stress, noise or glare. It is aggravated by the administration of vasoconstrictor agents and improved by vasodilators (Brazil and Friedman, 1956; Ostfeld, Reis and Wolff, 1957). A headache which is relieved by the taking of alcohol is almost invariably of the tension variety, whereas most vascular headaches become more severe. Muscle-contraction headache is usually relieved by aspirin or preparations which combine caffeine with analgesics, but it recurs after some hours. This may lead to repeated self-medication with subsequent risk of habituation and toxicity.

Physical examination

Formal neurological examination is usually normal, but signs of muscular overcontraction are found in the majority of patients. Some patients look the part, with deep wrinkles on face and forehead where time has etched their personality traits. The temporal and masseter muscles may stand out and twitch, and the hands may clench the chair

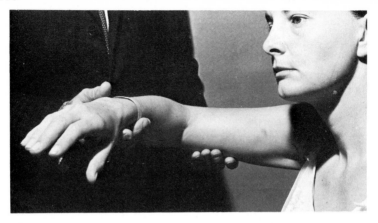

Figure 9.3. Testing the ability of a patient with tension headache to relax skeletal muscles at will. The patient is instructed to let the arm go loose in the examiner's hand as though it were resting on an armchair

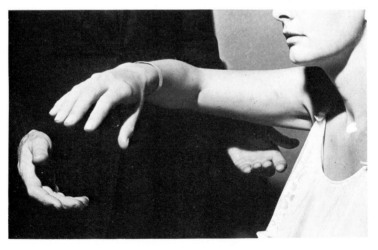

Figure 9.4. When the examiner's hand is removed, the patient's arm remains on the invisible armchair. The patient had been unaware that the arm was not completely relaxed

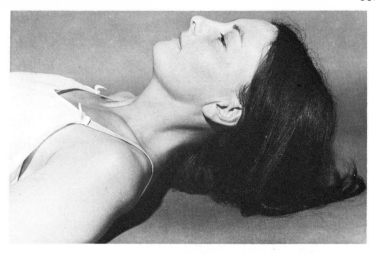

Figure 9.5. Difficulty in relaxing the neck muscles in a patient with tension headache. The examiner's hands have just been removed from a position where they were 'supporting' the patient's head. The neck muscles continued to contract so that the head remained elevated after the hands were withdrawn

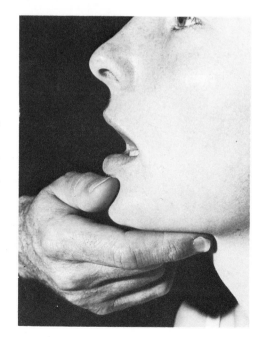

Figure 9.6. The ability to relax the jaw muscles can be tested by attempting to move the jaw rapidly up and down without displacing the head. In most patients with tension headache, the head moves with the jaw which is held rigidly

firmly or the fingers move restlessly during the interview. Other patients may have a bland appearance which is impassive due to muscular rigidity and rarely softens into a smile.

A simple test of the ability to relax is to lift the patient's arm up in one's hands and to tell the patient that he or she must imagine it is resting on an armchair (*Figure 9.3*). The aim is to let the limb go completely loose so that when the examiner's hands are removed the arm will flop lifelessly downwards to the patient's side. In fact, the vast majority of tension headache patients assure the examiner that the arm is completely relaxed and are surprised to find that it still rests on the imaginary armchair once the supporting hands are taken away (*Figure 9.4*). Similar to the 'armchair sign' is the 'invisible pillow'. A patient who is instructed to let the head loll back in the examiner's hands will frequently maintain the head rigidly in position above the couch (*Figure 9.5*) and can only put it down by a conscious voluntary extension movement of the neck. It should be possible to relax the legs so that they can be bent freely at the knees or rolled from side to side. Most patients with tension headache are quite unable to do this. It should be possible to let the jaw hang down so that it can be moved rapidly up and down through a small range by the examiner. Most tension headache patients hold the jaw so rigidly that the whole head moves with the mandible (*Figure 9.6*). Auscultation over the temporal muscles will confirm the presence of inappropriate contraction.

The constant driving from above of spinal mechanisms may induce such hyperactivity of stretch reflexes that the examiner may feel a sensation akin to the rigidity of Parkinson's disease on manipulating a joint through its range of movement. If the patient also has an exaggerated physiological tremor as part of an anxiety state, then the similarity to Parkinson's disease may be heightened by the superimposition of a cog-wheel effect on the increased muscle tone. Indeed, the mechanism is probably a functional or reversible overactivity of descending motor pathways which are thrown permanently into action in Parkinson's disease by anatomical and biochemical changes.

The elicitation of these physical signs of nervous tension is important not only for diagnosis but also to demonstrate to the patient that muscular hyperactivity is present, and to prepare the way for relaxation exercises as a part of treatment.

THE MECHANISM OF
MUSCLE-CONTRACTION HEADACHE

A constant factor in the production of tension headache appears to be the inability to relax the muscles of the face, scalp and neck, but not everyone with these characteristics develops headache. There is some additional element in the headache patient, which is not clearly understood, but which is probably hereditary. It may have to do with vascular reactivity in the muscles of scalp and neck, with the accumulation of pain-provoking substances in muscle, or with a central deficiency of inhibitory transmitter substances.

Psychological factors

Friedman, Von Storch and Merritt (1964), in an analysis of 1000 patients with tension headache, formed the impression that 'emotional factors are present in 100 per cent of these cases'. They considered that environmental demands of an economic, social, physical or intellectual nature beyond the capacity of the patient's personality produced somatic responses of which headache is the major symptom. Their patients demonstrated aggression, hostility and resentment against members of their family or persons who represent family figures.

Martin, Rome and Swenson (1967) studied 25 patients in detail and found that 22 described tension situations, usually involving dependence, sexuality and control of anger. These problems were exemplified by difficulty in leaving home, submission to a domineering spouse, broken marriages, impotence, frigidity, and a poor work record as well as specific emotional problems. The comment 'he's a pain in the neck' was often applied to a family member without realization of its literal application. Eight of the 25 patients had sexual problems such as premature ejaculation, dyspareunia and aversion to sexual intercourse. Nine patients were depressed. No fewer than 22 of the 25 patients had various psychosomatic disorders such as duodenal ulcer, vasomotor rhinitis, asthma, obesity and irritable bowel syndrome. Minnesota Multiphasic Personality Inventory tests showed no significant qualitative differences from the general population but the intensity of reaction was more with the emphasis on hypochondriasis, depression and hysteria. Another study (Gainotti, Cianchetti and Taramelli, 1972) compared 104 patients suffering from tension headache with 79 migrainous subjects. Symptoms of anxiety and depression were present in 95 per cent of the tension headache group compared with 54 per cent of the migraine patients.

Muscular contraction

Sainsbury and Gibson (1954) found that the electromyogram (EMG) recorded from the frontalis muscle was significantly greater in patients with anxiety states than in normal controls. At the time of recording, 7 patients who complained of headache or sensations of tightness or pressure in the head had significantly greater frontalis EMG activity than those without headache. In 1 patient whose headache increased during the recording, EMG activity increased. In 2 patients whose headaches progressively improved during the procedure, EMG activity declined. The association between muscle contraction and headache is therefore undeniable but it is still uncertain whether it is a primary or secondary phenomenon. Some patients may have some correctable source of excessive muscle contraction, such as an error of refraction, a latent strabismus, cervical spondylosis, or imbalance of the bite, throwing strain on one temporomandibular joint. Every (1960) has drawn attention to the nocturnal fang-sharpening movements of the jaw which occur during sleep as a manifestation of repressed aggression. The latter syndrome may be recognized by the association of chronic headache with pain in the temporomandibular joints and jaw muscles and a raw tender spot on the buccal mucosa opposite the posterior part of the upper gum, which results from excessive lateral movement of the mandible during sleep. This disorder responds to psychological management rather than measures directed solely to malocclusion.

CASE REPORT

Headache induced by jaw clenching.

A woman aged 52 years had suffered constant headaches for 22 years. The pain was a constant dull ache which spread across her eyes, nose, cheeks, temples, ears and upper teeth, which started when she married. The marriage was not a success and she found that she was always extremely tense and anxious. One of the symptoms of this was constant grinding of the teeth. She found herself doing it during the day and even woke herself up at night by the noise of her teeth clashing against one another. She would be dreaming that a train was coming through a station or that the roof was falling in and would awaken to find out that it was her own jaws clashing that had woken her up. She was aware of severe pain in the jaws at that time and her temporomandibular joints were so sore that she could not open her mouth to chew. She also noticed a dull ache like the present one. She left her husband after 7 years and has not married again. She continued to be a tense person and often noticed that she put her tongue between her teeth during the day to prevent jaw-clenching. Her pain was relieved by taking alcohol.

Vascular factors

Recordings of the pulsation from scalp arteries show that vascular reactions in tension headache are the reverse of those seen in migraine. Whereas the scalp vessels dilate in migraine attacks, the amplitude of their pulsation is reduced in tension headache (Tunis and Wolff, 1954). This suggests that patients are unable to 'summon up the blood' necessary to nourish the hyperactive scalp musculature. The small vessels of the conjunctiva have been examined and photographed during tension headache and have been seen to constrict as long as a frontal headache lasts (Ostfeld, Reis and Wolff, 1957). This unseemly vasoconstriction may be partly responsible for tension headache, since the pain becomes worse with vasoconstrictor agents such as noradrenaline and ergotamine, and is relieved temporarily by the inhalation of amyl nitrite or the administration of various vasodilator drugs, including alcohol (Brazil and Friedman, 1956; Ostfeld, Reis and Wolff, 1957). To test the vaso-constrictive hypothesis, a research group in New York injected a radio-active sodium preparation into the muscles at the back of the neck and checked its rate of clearance during severe occipital headache (Onel, Friedman and Grossman, 1961). Surprisingly, they found that clearance was greater than it was in headache-free periods. At first sight this appears to be evidence against constriction of muscular arteries, but this interpretation need not be correct, because the studies were made in patients with headache of fluctuating intensity when headache was severe, thus resembling the description of 'tension-vascular headache' rather than the milder pressure sensations of the usual muscle-contraction headache.

The possibility of a deficiency of mono-amine transmitters in the central nervous system playing a part in chronic tension headache was raised by a recent observation of Rolf, Wiele and Brune (1977). They found that morning blood samples taken from patients subject to frequent tension headache contained significantly less serotonin than samples taken from normal controls and from headache-free migraine subjects. No comparison has yet been made between tension headache patients with and without headache to see whether the low serotonin level is a reflection of the headache state as it is in migraine or whether it is a constant finding. It is also possible that chemical changes may take place either systemically, or locally in muscles or their vessels, which sensitize end-organs to pain perception. Most tension headaches respond readily, if temporarily, to aspirin. The intraperitoneal injection of aspirin in man will prevent the pain which is induced by the intra-peritoneal injection of bradykinin, whereas the same dose given intra-venously is ineffective (Lim *et al.*, 1967). This suggests that aspirin analgesia in man may be due to blockade of pain receptors at the periphery, and that pains which are responsive to aspirin may depend upon some chemical mediator such as bradykinin.

Central factors

The interpretation of sensory patterns may be different in the patient with 'muscle-contraction' headache. Many patients are introspective and have a low pain threshold in that they may complain of other uncomfortable sensations in various parts of the body. Sicuteri (1977) has postulated that the syndrome of 'non-organic central pain' (which includes the entity commonly described as muscle-contraction or tension headache) is caused by a failure of the normal mechanisms for the prevention of pain, the antinociceptive system. This in turn might be the result of a central deficiency in mono-amines or endorphins (polypeptides which are thought to act as inhibitory transmitters on pain pathways). The cause of pain, of the constriction of scalp arteries and conjunctival arterioles in tension headache, and of increased blood-flow in some patients with tension or tension-vascular headache still has to be elucidated, quite apart from the complex psychological tangle which may underlie the observable manifestations in the head and neck.

TREATMENT OF TENSION HEADACHE

Most patients suffering from chronic muscle-contraction headache suspect that they have a cerebral tumour or other serious intracranial disorder. The first step in treatment is to give patients a good hearing and careful examination, to give them confidence that their complaint is being taken seriously and that the doctor is not jumping to a facile conclusion in order to prescribe a tranquillizer and move on to the next patient. It is often advisable to support one's clinical opinion by arranging for an electroencephalogram, isotope scan and radiography of the skull and chest to provide for the patients some objective evidence that their fears are groundless.

The second step in treatment is to demonstrate that the scalp and facial muscles are indeed contracting for much of the time without reason. This can be achieved partly by questions at the end of history taking. Do your friends comment that you always look serious or worried? Do you find yourself clenching your jaws, grinding your teeth, making a tight fist with your hands? The answers to these questions can be quite surprising. Some patients have had to seek dental attention because their teeth are tender or chipped from unremitting pressure of their jaws (*Figure 9.7*). The author has had patients who had broken their dentures repeatedly by the same mechanism. Some state that they notice their fingers flexed firmly even on awakening from sleep.

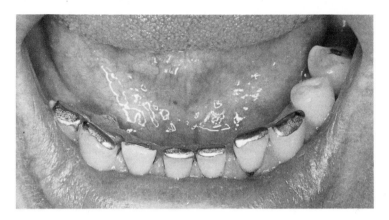

Figure 9.7. Dental restoration required by a patient because her habit of clenching her jaws had worn away the tooth enamel

The presence of unnecessary muscular contraction can be shown to the patient at the end of physical examination. Most are unable to relax the jaw muscles so that the jaw can be moved freely by the physician. They are unable to let the head loll back when the shoulders are supported since the neck muscles remain rigid. They cannot permit their elevated arm to fall limply to the couch when requested by the examiner.

Correction of various physical factors may be necessary to help patients reach their goal of muscular relaxation. Correction of a refractive error, or orthoptic treatment for a latent ocular imbalance, may remove the factor of eye-strain which sets up a pattern of wasteful muscle activity. Dental treatment may be important to open a closed bite, restore a chewing surface, or improve dentures so that the bite is evenly distributed. Cervical traction or manipulation may be useful if neck pain from degenerated intervertebral discs is triggering the tension headache.

The management of the patient with tension headache must of necessity be psychological, physiological (aimed at relaxation of the facial and scalp muscles) and often pharmacological as well.

Psychological management

It may be argued that all patients with muscle-contraction headache should be referred to a psychiatrist in the first instance. This is certainly the author's policy with any patient who shows signs of serious mental disturbance, but it is not practical for every tense patient to be seen by a psychiatrist, nor would it be desirable because many patients are resentful of the implication of mental illness. The majority can be managed by the doctor of first contact providing he or she has the time and interest to take a careful history and counsel the patient. Some patients will not admit to any problem or source of anxiety and may simply have a long-standing habit of muscle contraction in response to the ordinary pressures of everyday life. Others may have easily identifiable worries and anxieties concerned with their work or home life which may respond to sympathetic discussion. Some tension headaches clear up as soon as the patient goes on vacation. One woman told me that her symptoms mysteriously eased as soon as her husband went away on a business trip only to return as soon as he did. The man or woman whose spouse is disdaining, disaffected, drunk, drugged, debauched or otherwise despicable, lives with a constant provocation to headache which may be hard to remove by any amount of psychological counselling. Careful thought about the patient and his or her reactions to stress, combined with advice about relationships to others and adjustment of work pattern and life style will help to ease the patient's anxiety. The use of social agencies to provide support for those who are slowly losing the struggle for existence on their own is also part of the doctor's role in helping the patient to overcome the symptom of headache. Referral of an individual or couple for expert sexual counselling can often be very useful for, even in these enlightened and liberated times, there are many whose lives are lived in sexual ignorance or blighted by feelings of inadequacy, shame or guilt which are often lightened by confiding in their medical adviser.

Martin and Rome (1967) consider that anxiety is often a secondary response to anger in patients with muscle-contraction headaches and relates to multiple conflicts that are usually evident. They emphasize that a careful, unhurried history and an appreciation of the factors causing stress is essential for psychological management, which may require only 'a single corrective emotional experience', or may involve long-term psychotherapy or group therapy. Mitchell and White (1977) presented a detailed case-history of the management of a patient with tension headache by the teaching of 'social engineering skills' (modifying stress factors), self-control skills (coping with residual stress) and organizational skills (planning for the future). They point out that this form of 'behavioural self-management' is both economical and portable. 'People themselves are the best possible agents of their own behaviour change; they certainly have more frequent access to it than anyone else.'

The author's practice is to combine simple counselling at the first interview with an explanation of how the patient's emotional conflicts are translated into headache by muscular activity. This is then followed by some form of relaxation therapy, considered as physiological management.

Psysiological management

Relaxation exercises, usually modified from those described by Jacobsen (1938), have become generally accepted as the most direct means of overcoming the habitual overcontraction of muscles in tension headache. Warner and Lance (1975) combined relaxation therapy with some of the techniques of transcendental meditation in the treatment of 17 patients with chronic tension headache. Personal tuition was followed by the patient practising at home with the help of tape recordings of the instructor's voice. When the patients were followed up after 6 months, 4 were headache-free, 7 were subject to 1 to 4 headaches each month (instead of 12 to 30) and only 6 were unimproved. Only 3 required analgesics or tranquillizers whereas 14 were habitual users before relaxation therapy.

The use of feedback methods to guide the patient in controlling muscle activity and promoting relaxation has increased in recent years. Feedback from the electromyogram (EMG) of the frontal or temporal muscles has been the most popular method. The amplified EMG signal is played back to the patient through a loudspeaker or earphones, either directly or transformed into a clicking, humming or buzzing noise which varies in intensity in proportion to the integrated EMG activity. Budzynski *et al.* (1973) reported the result of a controlled trial in which the response of 6 patients treated by EMG feedback was compared with that of 6 patients treated by pseudofeedback' (sounds uncorrelated with muscle activity) and 6 untreated controls. Treatment consisted of sixteen 20-minute feedback sessions augmented by daily practice at home. They found that there was a significant decrease in muscle activity, headache and intake of analgesics and tranquillizers in the treated group but not in the other groups. Improvement was maintained after eighteen months by 3 patients who had responded well to the initial course of treatment. Another patient showed slight long-term improvement and 2 were lost to follow-up. The authors estimated that EMG activity can be reduced by 50 to 70 per cent with 3 to 6 sessions of training.

Feedback from the electroencephalogram (EEG) has been employed to alter the pattern of arousal (suppression of alpha rhythm and excessive fast activity) to one of relaxation with a well-developed alpha rhythm. Dominance of alpha rhythm caused a monitoring screen to turn blue and fast activity in the beta range produced a red colour. The subject was encouraged to relax until the blue colour appeared, for two sessions weekly for 5 weeks. By the fifth week of treatment, reduction in hours of headache averaged 80 per cent. A follow-up six months to three years later (Montgomery and Ehrisman, 1976) indicated that improvement was maintained.

There are probably many ways in which the patient can be made aware of muscular tension and ways of relieving it. Our own practice is to explain the relaxation process to the patients, then give them a simple instruction pamphlet which is reproduced at the end of this chapter. Some patients are seen by a psychologist attached to the Neurology Clinic for EMG biofeedback therapy while others are referred to physiotherapists who take a particular interest in relaxation therapy. This approach may be sufficient to relieve tension headache without any need for tranquillizing or antidepressant agents.

CASE REPORT

The following illustrates the relief of chronic tension headache by the use of relaxation exercises.

A school-teacher aged 49 years had been subject to headaches 4 or 5 days every week for 23 years. The sensation was described as a discomfort behind the forehead and eyes, which became more severe about once a month, when he felt mildly nauseated. There were no migrainous features about the headache, which came on at about midday and persisted through the afternoon, made worse by glare or concentration. He was a bachelor who had looked after his aged father until he died two years previously. He had no obvious problems but he stated he had a meticulous nature and people commented on his frowning, since he had always found it hard to relax. He was given a prescription for amitriptyline, and relaxation exercises were explained to him. He then returned to the country town where he lived and practised the exercises assiduously. The frequency of his headaches diminished to once a week or once a fortnight and he wrote to say that he had not had his prescription filled as he found that he remained virtually free of headaches as long as he continued his daily period of relaxation.

Pharmacological management

Ideally it should never be necessary to prescribe any medication in tension headache. Evaluation of any personal problem and helping the patient to overcome it, explanation of the mechanism of headache and the demonstration of muscular relaxation should be sufficient to prevent further headaches. Unfortunately, it does not work out like this, possibly because not enough is known about all the factors involved in the mechanism, and possibly because many patients are quite unable to relax even when shown how to do so.

In 1964, a trial was undertaken at our clinic to assess the effect of various drugs on 280 patients who were subject to tension headache for at least 10 days of each month (Lance and Curran, 1964). The majority (239) of these patients experienced headaches daily. The headaches had been present for over 5 years in 211 patients and for more than 20 years in 111 patients. It was found that the use of sedatives alone (usually amylobarbitone), vasodilator drugs alone or a combination of the two, gave a response which was no different on statistical analysis from that to placebo. The muscle-relaxing drug, orphenadrine, and the migraine prophylactic drug, methysergide, were of no benefit. Improvement was obtained with the antidepressants amitriptyline (Elavil, Laroxyl, Tryptanol, Tryptizol) and imipramine (Tofranil) as well as with the tranquillizing agents chlordiazepoxide (Librium) and diazepam (Valium) and Bellergal (a proprietary product containing ergotamine tartrate 0.3 mg, phenobarbitone 20 mg, and belladonna alkaloids 0.1 mg). A double-blind controlled cross-over trial was carried out with amitriptyline, which confirmed that its action did not depend upon any placebo effect. Of the patients starting the trial, 47 did not report to the clinic again after a trial of only one drug. Of the 233 who were given a number of preparations, 74 per cent improved on one or other form of medication.

As a result of this trial it has been my practice to give patients a trial period of 1 month on diazepam, 5 mg three times daily, if they are simply tense and anxious, or to use amitriptyline, 25 mg three times daily, if they are also depressed. In either instance, the patient is recommended to take one-half tablet three times daily for the first few days, since diazepam may cause drowsiness and ataxia in some people and amitriptyline may produce drowsiness, tremor, dryness of the mouth and gain in weight. It is advisable not to give amitriptyline to patients with glaucoma because of its atropine-like side-effects. Amitriptyline is not only useful in depressed patients. Of the 98 patients treated with amitriptyline in our clinical trial, 58 improved substantially, and only 18 of these had symptoms of depression. Some 7 per cent of patients are unable to tolerate amitriptyline, but it is worth a trial in any patient with chronic headache. It may be an advantage to give the full daily dosage of amitriptyline before the patient retires for the night. This may prevent drowsiness during the day, help insomnia, and does not interfere with the long-term antidepressant action. Patients who respond satisfactorily lose their headaches or notice substantial improvement from 2 to 10 days after starting treatment and it is then suggested that they continue treatment for at least 6 months and then wean off the medication slowly over a period of 2 to 3 months. If headaches return after treatment is stopped they usually recur after 2 to 14 days.

PSYCHOGENIC HEADACHE

The term 'psychogenic headache' is used to describe the association of headache with florid psychiatric disturbance such as acute depression, schizophrenia or hysteria. Headache may be incorporated into the delusional system of such patients. There is no way in which any mechanism can be postulated for such headaches incorporating peripheral pain pathways. The headache is a concept of disordered thought processes and appears or disappears with the mental state which engendered it.

CASE REPORT

The following presents a case of headache in paranoid schizophrenia.
A man aged 43 years had suffered from constant bilateral headache, '7 days a week and 24 hours a day' for the past 7 years. He had been a champion boxer in earlier days and considered that his frontal lobes had been damaged by boxing injuries. He stated that he had been 'bashed up by the underworld' thousands of times and that his recent head injuries had brought back memories of head injuries 20 years ago. He said that the underworld, under the leadership of a prominent judge, had been squirting cyanide through water pistols into his bedroom and placing rubber masks over his head. He felt 'boiled up' and 'filled with hate' and had the sensation of an ulcer in his head. His present headache was attributed to cyanide administered per rectum while he was unconscious from a pellet-gun wound.

APPENDIX

Relaxation exercises: instructions issued to patients with tension or tension-vascular headaches

What has muscle contraction to do with headache?

The blood vessels and nerve fibres of the scalp lie in muscle. Place your fingers on each temple and clench your jaw. You will feel the muscle belly of the temporal muscle swell as it contracts. Let the jaw go loose and the muscle becomes flat again. Many people contract these muscles all day without realizing it so they are working continuously, which sets up a constant dull ache in the temples. The vessels which run through the muscles often constrict while the muscle is contracting. During sleep the muscles may relax and the vessels dilate so that a person may wake in the middle of the night or the early morning with a throbbing headache in the temples. Some others may grind or clash their teeth at night during sleep and may therefore wake up with aching jaws and a raw tender spot on their upper gum caused by sideways movement of the jaw during sleep. Overcontraction of the jaw muscles is very common in tense or anxious people, who often do not realize that their muscles are not relaxed.

Do you feel the jaw muscles aching at the end of the day, or after an unpleasant or difficult conversation, or after an argument? Do you feel an ache in one or both temples at these times or wake up with a headache in this area? If the headache is in one temple only, check your bite to see if you chew equally and evenly on both sides and can move the jaw freely from side to side. If you have back teeth missing on one side or the other, the strain of chewing is thrown on to the other side which causes an ache in the hinge-joint of the jaw and in the temple. If this is the case you should see your dentist about balancing the bite, as this can be a very important factor in excessive jaw-clenching.

Just as chronic jaw-clenching is a common cause of aching in the temples, chronic frowning is a common cause of pain in the forehead. Do others say to you that you frown a lot or look worried most of the time? This can be an indication that you are using your scalp muscles without being aware of it.

Pain in the neck can also result from muscle contraction. Some people walk about holding their neck stiffly as though it were a solid block of wood. This may be an attempt to protect the neck because of the sensation of grating in the neck on movement or the discovery on x-ray that some of the discs in the neck have degenerated. Disc degeneration is quite common even in young people and is almost universal in older age groups. If there has been a whip-lash injury to the neck or attention is drawn to the neck in any way, the muscles may contract to splint the neck and a vicious cycle is set up of pain leading to muscle spasm which leads to more pain.

Muscle-contraction or tension headache is usually a constant tight pressing feeling in the forehead, temples or back of the head and may spread all around the head 'like a tight band'. Because the scalp muscles are linked together by a sheet of strong tissue which passes over the skull, muscle contraction may also cause the feeling of pressure on top of the head. Sharp jabbing pains may also be felt because scalp nerves are compressed by muscle contraction.

Overcontraction of muscle is a faulty habit which develops over the years and often starts in childhood. About 1 in 7 of patients with tension headache can remember having similar headaches under the age of 10 years. It may be associated with mental tension and anxiety but may have become an automatic reaction which continues even when there are no obvious problems of any sort.

Are you able to relax?

The most natural form of treatment is to train the muscles of the body to relax and the first step is to realize that you are not as relaxed as you think you are.

Try these simple tests.

(1) Sit in a chair and lean back. Ask someone to lift your arm in the air in a comfortable position as though it were resting on the side of an arm-chair. Take your time and relax completely. Then ask your friend to take away his hands which have been supporting your arm. When the supporting hands are taken away, what does your arm do?

If it flops lifelessly downwards, you are indeed relaxed.

If it stays in the air, or you move it slowly downwards, you are not relaxed. Your muscles are contracting continuously *without you realizing it*.

(2) Lie on a bed or couch with your head on a pillow and try to relax completely. When you consider that you have achieved this, ask your accomplice to pull the pillow away from under your head. Does your head drop limply on to the bed?

Or does it stay poised in mid-air as though the pillow was still there?

If you are still holding your head in the air above an invisible pillow, your muscles must be contracting *without you realizing it.*

Once you have acknowledged that excessive muscle contraction is playing a part in the aching of your head or neck, and that you do not really know whether the muscles are contracting or not, you are ready to start relaxation exercises.

Paradoxically, you cannot relax about relaxing. It is not a passive process. It is no use saying to someone 'relax' and imagine that they can do it without further thought. You cannot say to yourself 'relax' and then do it unless you have carefully practised the art of 'switching off' the nerve supply to the muscles. This is a voluntary action as deliberate as turning off a light switch and must be practised until it can be done at will and done rapidly.

At first it is necessary to set aside at least ten minutes night and morning for the exercises. It is a great help to have someone with you in the early stages to ensure that you are completely relaxed when you think you are. This person will be referred to below as the 'assistant'. It is obviously a great advantage if the assistant can be a trained physiotherapist or occupational therapist but this is not always practicable and a well-motivated husband or wife, relative or friend can be of enormous value in ensuring that the exercises are performed conscientiously and that relaxation is practised until it becomes complete.

The sequence of relaxation exercises

Lie down on a firm surface such as a carpeted floor. A bed with an inner spring mattress will do, but not one with a soft, sagging mattress. A pillow can be used to support the head at first but may be discarded later as relaxation becomes easier. For the first few sessions only a short-sleeved shirt and shorts should be worn so that muscle contraction can be seen as well as felt. Lie on the back with the legs slightly separated and the arms comfortably flexed at the elbow so that the elbows are by the sides with the hands resting on the body. Various muscles will be contracted and relaxed in turn.

1. *Legs.*   Contract the leg muscles so that the legs become rigid pillars. The muscle bellies will be seen to stand out as the muscles contract. Concentrate on the sensation set up by the muscles contracting, and the feeling of tension in them. Then, suddenly and deliberately, 'switch off the power supply' so that the

muscles become limp. Concentrate on whether any sensation is coming from the muscles now. Are they completely relaxed? At this point it is helpful for an assistant to put his hand behind the subject's knees and lift them up sharply to see if the leg is completely floppy and that the muscles do not contract again as soon as the limb is moved passively. If they are not completely relaxed, or if they contract again when the limb is touched or moved, the sequence should be repeated.

Many people only half relax on the first few attempts. This can be detected by watching the muscles closely. After the first relaxation, the muscle bellies are not as prominent as they were but there may be some contraction remaining. Try again to 'switch off' and this second attempt may be rewarded by seeing the muscle become completely flaccid. The legs may then be bent at the knee by the assistant, moved about, or rolled backwards and forwards with the feet flailing 'like a rag doll'. This sequence may be completed by lifting one leg, letting it drop downwards like an inanimate object, then doing the same with the other.

2. *Arms.* Brace the arms so that the elbows are forced downwards on the couch (or on the assistant's hand if he is checking the degree of relaxation). The arms are held rigidly and the muscle contraction is suddenly stopped so that the arms become limp and lifeless. The assistant should then be able to bounce the elbow up and down without any resistance being offered. This sequence should be repeated until the subject is aware of the sensation of muscle contraction and the contrast with the feeling of relaxation, and the assistant is satisfied that the arm becomes truly flaccid.

3. *Neck.* Lift the head from the pillow and then allow it to drop backwards. The assistant may provide resistance by pressing on the forehead until the subject feels the contraction of the muscles in the front of the neck. When the head is dropped backwards, the assistant can rock it gently to and fro to make certain that there is no residual activity in the muscles. Now push the head backwards into the pillow and register the sensation of contraction of the muscles in the back of the neck. Stop the contraction suddenly so that the head may be rotated freely on the neck by the assistant. Repeat this until relaxation is satisfactory.

4. *Forehead.* Frown upwards so that the brow is furrowed. If there is difficulty in doing this, look upwards as far as the eyes will move and the forehead will become creased. Again, feel the sensation of tension in the muscles, then close the eyes and let the forehead muscles relax. The assistant can detect the presence

or absence of contraction by seeing whether the skin of the forehead moves freely with his hand.

5. *Eyes.*   Screw the eyes up tightly and become aware of the sensation of tension, then relax the muscles and lie with the eyes closed lightly. Make sure that there is no trembling or flickering of the closed eyelids and that the eye muscles feel entirely relaxed.

6. *Jaw.*   Clench the jaw firmly and concentrate on feeling the sense of tightness in the temples as well as in the jaw itself. Then switch off and let the jaw fall open. Push the jaw open, perhaps against the pressure of the assistant's hand, then relax completely. Move the jaw sideways to the right as far as it will go and experience the sensation which this gives to the jaw and temple before relaxing. Then do the same to the left. Complete the sequence by clenching the jaw firmly again, and let the jaw drop open loosely. The assistant should then be able to hold the tip of the jaw with his fingers and waggle the jaw up and down rapidly without any opposition from the jaw muscles.

This is the hardest of all relaxation procedures to achieve and you must not be disappointed if you are unsuccessful on the first occasion. It may require repeated practice to enable the jaw muscles to cease all activity so that the jaw may be moved easily by the assistant. It is most important that you persevere until you accomplish this because overcontraction of jaw muscles is the most common factor in tension headache and the 'switching-off' process must be thoroughly learned.

7. *Whole body relaxation.*   Once you are able to relax the legs, arms, neck, forehead, eye and jaw muscles in order, lie for five minutes with all muscles relaxed. Once you have achieved total relaxation, the process becomes negative rather than positive. In other words, you permit natural relaxation to continue rather than willing yourself to relax actively. At this stage, it is helpful to think of some beautiful and tranquil scene, to imagine yourself lying on a grassy bank on a warm summer's day with the drowsy sounds of summer in the background. Everyone has some particular sound he or she associates with peace and tranquillity. It may be the rippling of a trout stream, the humming of bees, the song of birds, the soughing of wind in the trees, or distant music. Choose your own theme and your own mental picture and live in that scene for a few minutes. As you do so, feel the sensation of heaviness creep over your legs, trunk and arms, then spread to your neck and head, eyes and face. Lie completely inert, with all muscles relaxed, a feeling of heaviness throughout

the body and a pleasant scene pictured in the mind. Feel the
sensation of freedom in the mind and in the head. This can
become a permanent freedom if your muscles obey you all the
time as well as they do at that moment.

8. *After relaxation exercises are finished.* The final and most
important step is to carry the art of relaxation into your everyday life. Watch the way you stand, the way you sit, the way in
which you speak on the telephone, talk to people, write, type or
perform any other activity of a typical day. Check that all the
muscles which are not essential to the task of the moment are
in a state of relaxation. You can handle any situation, irrespective of the degree of mental stress, without physical tension once
you become accustomed to the idea. You actually perform more
efficiently if you tackle any problem in an orderly fashion without excessive and useless muscle contraction. If you notice any
warning sensations of tension in the scalp, jaw or neck muscles,
you must pause a moment to ensure that these muscles are
'switched off' in the manner you have practised. In this way you
will finish the day feeling much fresher and with much less
chance of headache making your day a misery.

9. *Keep practising.* There is no point in performing the exercise
routine religiously for a week and then forgetting the whole
thing. If you do, unless you are a very exceptional person, the old
habits of muscle contraction will assert themselves again. Keep
practising, stay relaxed and free yourself from headache.

REFERENCES

Brazil, P. and Friedman, A.P. (1956). Craniovascular studies in headache. A
report and analysis of pulse volume tracings. *Neurology, Minneap.* 6, 96

Budzynski, T.H. Stoyva, J.M., Adler, C.S. and Mullaney, D.J. (1973). EMG
biofeedback and tension headache: a controlled outcome study. *Psychosom.
Med.* 35, 484

Every, R.G. (1960). The significance of extreme mandibular movement. *Lancet*
2, 37

Friedman, A.P., Von Storch, T.J.C. and Merritt, H.H. (1964). Migraine and tension
headaches. A clinical study of two thousand cases. *Neurology* 4, 773

Gainotti, G., Cianchetti, C. and Taramelli, M. (1972). Anxiety, level and psycho-
dynamic mechanisms in medical headaches. *Res. clin. Stud. Headache (Karger/
Basel)* 3, 182

Jacobsen, E. (1938). *Progressive Relaxation.* Illinois: University of Chicago Press

Lance, J.W. and Anthony, M. (1966). Some clinical aspects of migraine. *Archs
Neurol.* 15, 356

Lance, J.W. and Curran, D.A. (1964). Treatment of chronic tension headache.
Lancet 1, 1236

Lance, J.W., Curran, D.A. and Anthony, M. (1965). Investigations into the mechanism and treatment of chronic headache. *Med. J. Aust.* **2**, 909

Lim, R.K.S., Miller, D.G., Guzman, F., Rodgers, D.W., Rogers, R.W., Wang, S.K., Chao, P.Y. and Shih, T.Y. (1967). Pain and analgesia evaluated by the intraperitoneal bradykinin-evoked pain method in man. *Clin. Pharmac. Ther.* **8**, 521

McKenzie, R.E., Ehrisman, W.J., Montgomery, P.S. and Barnes, R.H. (1974). The treatment of headache by means of electroencephalographic biofeedback. *Headache* **13**, 164

Martin, M.J. and Rome, H.P. (1967). Muscle-contraction headache: therapeutic aspects. *Res. clin Stud. Headache (Karger/Basel)* **1**, 205

Martin, M.J., Rome, H.P. and Swenson, W.M. (1967). Muscle-contraction headache: a psychiatric review. *Res. clin. Stud. Headache (Karger/Basel)* **1**, 184

Mitchell, K.R. and White, R.G. (1977). Self-management of tension headaches: a case study. *J. Behav. Ther. Exp. Psychiat.* In press

Montgomery, P.S. and Ehrisman, W.J. (1976). Biofeedback-alleviated headaches: a follow-up. *Headache* **16**, 64

Onel, Y., Friedman, A.P. and Grossman, J. (1961). Muscle blood flow studies in muscle-contraction headache. *Neurology, Minneap.* **11**, 935

Ostfeld, A.M. Reis, D.J. and Wolff, H.G. (1957). Studies on headache: bulbar conjunctival ischaemia and muscle-contraction headache. *Archs Neurol. Psychiat., Chicago* **77**, 113

Rolf, L.H., Wiele, G. and Brune, G.G. (1977). Serotonin in platelets of patients with migraine and muscle-contraction headache. *Excerpta med.* **427**, 11–12

Sainsbury, P. and Gibson, J.G. (1954). Symptoms of anxiety and tension and the accompanying physiological changes in the muscular system. *J. Neurol. Neurosurg. Psychiat.* **17**, 216

Sicuteri, F. (1977). Monoamine supersensitivity in non-organic central pain (idiopathic headache). *Excerpta med.* **427**, 194

Tunis, M.M. and Wolff, H.G. (1954). Studies on headache. Cranial artery vasoconstriction and muscle-contraction headache. *Archs Neurol. Psychiat., Chicago,* **71**, 425

Warner, G. and Lance, J.W. (1975) Relaxation therapy in migraine and chronic tension headache. *Med. J. Aust.* **1**, 298

Ten

Migraine

CLINICAL FEATURES

Prevalence

Migraine is a common disorder, but just how common has been a subject of dispute in the past. One of the main difficulties in all surveys has been the definition of migraine because of the wide variation in the nature, frequency and severity of attacks. Some individuals who have had only one or two attacks of migraine in their lives could hardly be included as 'sufferers from migraine'. On the other hand, there are patients who have less severe forms of headache, particularly of the tension variety, who are anxious to upgrade their symptoms and acquire the prestige of being a migraineur, who might unwittingly inflate the result of any survey. A survey of neurological disease in the English city of Carlisle (Brewis *et al.*, 1966) found that 3.3 per cent of the community was subject to migraine and that another 3 per cent complained of other forms of chronic headache which were sufficiently frequent and severe to cause loss of time from work or school.

Bille (1962) studied a group of almost 9 000 Swedish children and found that the prevalence increased during childhood from 1 per cent at the age of 6 years to 5 per cent at the age of 11 years. Of the migrainous children, 42 per cent were subject to one or more attacks each month which were sufficiently severe to prevent the child from carrying on with his or her usual occupation. There was no significant difference in the hours lost from school by boys with migraine than by boys who did not suffer from headache. However, migrainous girls lost a mean of 50 hours from school per term, compared with 27 hours for girls not subject to headache.

Dalsgaard-Nielsen (1970) reported a higher incidence than Bille for

130

each age group in 2 027 Danish children, and found that the prevalence in women reached 19 per cent by the age of 40. This figure is in agreement with Waters and O'Connor (1970), who calculated that 19 per cent of 2 933 women between the ages of 20 and 64 years in a region of Wales suffered from migraine. Of 56 migrainous women interviewed, only 13 (23 per cent) had consulted a doctor for their headaches in the previous year and 26 (46 per cent) said that they had never seen a doctor at any time in their lives for headache.

The peak incidence of migraine is reached in women during the reproductive years of life and then declines as age advances. Whitty and Hockaday (1968) obtained information about 92 patients who had attended a neurology clinic 14 years before. Attacks had ceased in 27 patients and were less severe in 44. Of the 18 patients over the age of 64 only 9 were still subject to migraine. Walker (1959) studied 5 785 records from a general practice in the Liverpool area of England and interviewed patients with a history of recurrent headache. A past or present history of migraine was obtained in 4·85 per cent of patients. Walker analysed the data in 150 migrainous patients over the age of 30 and found that 20 of 38 males and 84 of 112 females were subject to attacks more often than once each month. Sweetnam (1961) found that only one-third of the patients diagnosed as having migraine were referred to a neurologist. It is clear that migraine is a major source of morbidity in the community and is managed mainly by the general practitioner.

Definition of the migraine syndrome

The term migraine is of French origin and comes from the Greek 'hemicrania' like the old English word 'megrim'. The classical concept of migraine is that of a paroxysmal disturbance of cerebral function associated with unilateral headache and vomiting. The definition of migraine has widened in recent years to include bilateral headaches. It is not unusual for patients to experience pain over the entire head with the same accompaniments as their unilateral attacks. Other patients may have bilateral or unilateral headaches, which are typical of migraine in their sudden onset and severity and association with nausea and photophobia, but which are not preceded by visual or other neurological symptoms. Gowers (1893) pointed out that the same patients may have simple headaches at one period of their life and more complex symptoms at another time.

> The simple headaches have the same characters and occur under the same causal conditions of heredity, etc., as those in which there are in addition other sensory symptoms.

To test the validity of this extension of the definition of migraine, a survey was done at the Northcott Neurological Centre in Sydney of 290 patients who had been diagnosed as having migraine (Selby and Lance, 1960).

Classical migrainous symptoms such as aphasia, paraesthesiae and visual disturbances (ranging from flashing lights in front of the eyes through zig-zag fortification spectra to scotomas and hemianopia) occurred in 101 of these patients, preceding the headache in 49 and concurrently with the headache in 52. These cardinal symptoms of migraine were associated with bilateral headaches as often as with hemicrania. There was no significant difference in the frequency of vomiting, photophobia, scalp tenderness or other parameters of migraine between those with unilateral or bilateral headaches, and the percentage with a family history of migraine was the same in both groups. The headaches of the 189 patients who were not subject to focal neurological symptoms were otherwise typical of migraine.

The Research Group on Migraine and Headache of the World Federation of Neurology agreed on the following definition of migraine.

Migraine is a familiar disorder characterized by recurrent attacks of headache widely variable in intensity, frequency and duration. Attacks are commonly unilateral and are usually associated with anorexia, nausea and vomiting. In some cases they are preceded by, or associated with, neurological and mood disturbances.

All the above characteristics are not necessarily present in each attack or in each patient. Conditions which are generally accepted as falling within the above definition are as follows:

> *Classic migraine,* in which headache is preceded or accompanied by transient focal neurological phenomena, for example, visual, sensory or speech disturbance.
> *Non-classic migraine*, which is not associated with sharply defined focal neurological disturbances. This is the more common variety encountered.

Conditions which may fall within the category of migraine were listed by the Research Group on Headache as follows:

> *Cluster headache*: (synonyms: 'Harris' ciliary or migrainous neuralgia', 'Horton's histaminic cephalgia'.) This condition is considered by the author to be an entity distinct from migraine for reasons presented in Chapter 13.
> *Facial migraine*: (synonym: 'lower-half headache'.) Unilateral episodic facial pain associated with symptoms suggestive either of migraine or of cluster headache.
> *Ophthalmoplegic migraine*: episodic migraine-like attacks associated

with objective evidence of paresis of the extra-ocular muscles, usually those supplied by the third nerve, often outlasting the headache. A structural abnormality must be excluded before this diagnosis is made.

Hemiplegic migraine: a rare condition which may exhibit a dominant inheritance, characterized by episodic migrainous attacks associated with hemiplegia outlasting the headache.

To this list we should add the variation of *'vertebrobasilar migraine'*, described by Bickerstaff (1961a), in which brainstem symptoms, such as vertigo and ataxia, are associated with visual disturbance and an increased tendency to faint at the time of the migraine attack. The syndrome is thought to be caused by the constriction of the basilar and posterior cerebral arteries, and the fainting to result from ischaemia of the reticular formation. In *retinal migraine* loss of vision is limited to one eye. The term *complicated migraine* is used for those patients who are left with a persisting neurological deficit after a migraine attack.

Varieties of migraine

The Ad Hoc Committee on Classification of Headache considered those patients with characteristic sensory, motor or visual prodromes as 'classic' migraine and those without any focal neurological disturbance as 'common migraine'. This classification demarcates both ends of the spectrum but there are some patients whose headaches are difficult to classify into one group or the other because the only neurological symptoms may be vertigo, dysarthria or loss of concentration. These symptoms are almost certainly caused by the same intracranial process that is responsible for scintillating scotomas, but would not be accepted by many as criteria for 'classic migraine'. Other patients have headaches accompanied by symptoms of varying complexity so that their manifestations slide in and out of the criteria of classic migraine from episode to episode. The life history of a patient with migraine often illustrates this point. It is not uncommon for migraine to start with vomiting attacks in early childhood, to which headache may be added after some years. In later childhood the headache may become the main source of complaint and vomiting of secondary importance. As puberty is approached the classic prodromes may become superadded so that each headache is preceded by zig-zag fortification spectra or other symptoms. In middle age, vomiting may be deleted from the syndrome. At any stage of life, migrainous patients may be liable to episodes of focal neurological disturbance without headache or vomiting which are called *migraine equivalents*.

CASE REPORT

The following illustrates a case of migraine equivalent.

A university lecturer and statistician, aged 52 years, with a family history of migraine, suffered from attacks of classic migraine from the ages of 17 to 23 years. He was then free from all symptoms for 10 years, but at the age of 33 years a new symptom complex appeared without headaches. The attack would begin with acute blurring of vision for 3 or 4 minutes followed by distressing sensations of circles, lines and zig-zags dancing in front of his eyes. The attack was accompanied by nausea, giddiness and photophobia and ceased after 30 minutes, leaving him exhausted.

In view of the wide variation in clinical symptoms, it is remarkable that there is usually little difficulty in the diagnosis of migraine, the reason being the repetitive paroxysmal nature of the disorder. Difficulty arises when the frequency of attacks is such that migraine recurs almost daily or where migraine is superimposed upon daily tension headache. In both instances it may be difficult to sort out the vascular component from the background of nervous tension or depression.

Some varieties of migraine are sufficiently distinctive to warrant consideration as separate subgroups. The pain of migraine may involve one side of the face rather than the head and the condition is then called *facial migraine* or lower-half headache.

Facial migraine is unilateral and usually starts in the palate or angle of the nose, spreads to the cheek, ear or neck, and may radiate upwards to involve the territory characteristic of cluster headache. It is distinguished from cluster headache by the longer duration of lower-half headaches, which last for more than 4 hours and may last several days, by the absence of bouts of headache alternating with periods of freedom, and by its association with typical migrainous features such as gastro-intestinal disturbance. The management is essentially the same as that of migraine.

CASE REPORT

The following is a case of lower-half headache presenting in a patient with a past history of migraine.

A woman aged 34 years had been subject to bilateral throbbing headaches, associated with nausea, vomiting, photophobia and scalp tenderness, between the ages of 3 and 20 years. These attacks recurred about twice a month and lasted for 2 days at a time. She was completely free of headache from the age of 20 years until she reached the age of 30 years, when she experienced a different kind of headache. This started in the left cheek, spread to the left ear, the angle of the jaw, and then radiated down that side of the neck. She became nauseated with the pain but did not vomit. She noticed flashes of light in front of the left eye 'like little stars' as well as tingling in the left arm, which felt unnaturally light, for half an hour at the beginning of each attack. As the pain increased, the left side of her face became puffy, the left eye watered and light hurt her eyes. The left ear ached with the headache and she heard a buzzing noise in that ear. The episodes were brought on by alcoholic drinks and relieved partly by cold compresses. Her mother and her sister suffered from typical migraine. The attacks recurred two or three times each month, lasting for 2 to 3 days at a time, until she was placed on methysergide 2 mg, three times daily, which reduced the frequency of attacks to one in 3 months, and this attack lasted for 1 day only.

In another form, commonly running in families, unilateral weakness may be a consistent and dramatic example of focal neurological deficit accompanying migraine, and it has therefore been called *familial hemiplegic migraine* (Bradshaw and Parsons, 1965; Whitty, 1953). Hemiparesis is not necessarily contralateral to the side of the headache.

CASE REPORT

The following illustrates the problem of a family with 'hemiplegic migraine'.

A man aged 49 years has been subject to bouts of numbness and paralysis of one side of the body (usually the right) since the age of 17 years, which recur every 3 months or so. He feels full of energy and in unusually good spirits for an hour or so before the attack and can then predict that one is about to start. Numbness and weakness creep up from his hand to his shoulder and then move up his leg. After half an hour the right side of his face is affected and he is unable to speak. An hour after the onset he develops a severe left-sided throbbing headache which lasts for several hours. More severe attacks are associated with vomiting, confusion and a stuporous condition which may last for several days. His father had similar attacks all his life, characterized by right-sided weakness. Two out of the patient's 6 children are affected. Peter, aged 13 years, has had 4 attacks of headache with right hemiparesis. Anthony, aged 11 years, has had 4 episodes of left-sided headache and left hemiparesis over the last 5 years.

The persistent recurrence of double vision with migraine, associated with signs of paresis of some of the muscles responsible for eye movement, has been termed *ophthalmoplegic migraine* (Bickerstaff, 1964).

The third nerve is most commonly affected with the development of ptosis, a dilated pupil, and restricted movement of the eyes in all directions except lateral gaze. The condition must be distinguished from compression of the third nerve by aneurysm or other space-occupying lesion, and diagnosis can only be made after prolonged observation of the patient and exclusion of other conditions by carotid angiography.

CASE REPORT

The following illustrates a case of ophthalmoplegic migraine.

A man aged 60 years had been subject to frequent attacks of vomiting all his childhood since the age of 2 years. In late childhood, the episodes were associated with headache behind the left eye and photophobia. From the age of 14 years, the headaches recurred at intervals of 2 weeks, the left eyelid drooped at the onset of the attack and the left pupil was seen to dilate at this time. At the age of 17 years, the left eye deviated outwards with each attack and one year later it remained permanently in the abducted position. Ptosis recurred intermittently with further headaches but persisted between attacks from the age of 19 years. He continued to have left-sided headaches once each fortnight throughout his life. One brother suffered from frequent headaches without vomiting but there was no definite family history of migraine. Apart from the left third nerve palsy, no abnormality was found on examination. No intracranial bruit could be heard. Electroencephalography and a left carotid arteriogram were normal.

If visual hallucinations and scotomas are limited to one eye rather than one half field, then the term *retinal migraine* may be employed.

CASE REPORT

The following illustrates a case of 'retinal migraine'.

A flying instructor, aged 33 years, without a family history of migraine, developed attacks which started with a 'starry feeling' in front of the left eye. He then saw bright lights 'like silver paper' which lasted for approximately 30 seconds. Vision was then partially lost or completely lost in the left eye for a period of 5 minutes and the pupil was dilated during this time. The amblyopia then resolved, leaving a dull ache behind the left eye. He had experienced 8 attacks of this sort in a period of 2 years. Radiography of the skull, an EEG and a left carotid angiogram were normal.

If the brainstem and cerebellum are particularly affected by the vasoconstrictive phase, the syndrome is called *vertebrobasilar* migraine which will be considered further under the heading of Focal Neurological Symptoms and Signs.

Sex and age distribution

Migraine is much more common in women, who comprised 60 per cent of one series of 500 cases (Selby and Lance, 1960) and 75 per cent of another 500 cases (Lance and Anthony, 1971) which the author had the opportunity to analyse personally.

The first attack of migraine is experienced at the age of 10 years or younger by 25 per cent of patients (*see Figures 9.1* and *10.2*). One patient suffered his first episode at the age of 18 months. It is rare for migraine to make its appearance after the age of 45 years, but the author recalls 1 patient in whom typical migraine started at the age of 60 years. Migraine may be a lifelong complaint. The duration of headache at the time of seeking treatment in one personal series is shown in *Figure 9.2*.

Family history

When a family history includes only parents and siblings, 46 per cent of migrainous patients have a family history of migraine, compared with 18 per cent of patients suffering from typical tension headache who were used as a control group (Lance and Anthony, 1971). If grandparents are included as well, 55 per cent of patients have a positive family history (Selby and Lance, 1960). From a study of 832 offspring of 119 patients, Wolff (1972) concluded that migraine was inherited, probably through a recessive gene with a penetrance of approximately 70 per cent. Some families, however, clearly illustrate a dominant inheritance.

The migraine personality

Bo Bille (1962) compared personality characteristics of migrainous school-children with those of their fellows. There was no demonstrable difference in social class, intelligence or ambition, or in such symptoms as nervous tics, nail-biting or nocturnal enuresis. There was a higher incidence of sleep disturbances and 'night terrors', temper tantrums, recurrent abdominal pains and motion sickness among the migrainous children. The migraine group gave a slower performance in sensorimotor tests but with less errors than the control group. They were more fearful, tense, sensitive and vulnerable to frustration. They were tidier and less physically enduring than their non-migrainous counterparts. Waters (1975) also found that there was no correlation between intelligence or social class in the prevalence of migraine but that the more intelligent patients and those of higher social class consulted a doctor more frequently. The migraine patient is not subject to stress more often than those in a control group but reacts more to such stress (Henryk-Gutt and Rees, 1973). In an analysis of 500 migrainous patients (Selby and Lance, 1960), 23 per cent exhibited obsessional trends, being unnecessarily tidy or house-proud and in the habit of double-checking their actions. Some keep meticulous records of their headaches (*Figure 10.1*) which can be very helpful to their medical advisers as well as reflecting on their own industrious personality.

Relationship to epilepsy, allergy and childhood vomiting attacks

Many reports in the past have linked migraine with epilepsy, allergic disorders (asthma, hay fever, hives and eczema) and cyclical vomiting or 'bilious attacks' in childhood. Any uncontrolled observation is suspect because a migrainous patient is more likely to be referred for investigation if suffering from an associated illness, and the allergist, neurologist, psychiatrist or other specialist may receive a biased sample because of his particular interest. To obviate this, 100 patients with typical daily muscle-contraction headache were used as a control group to compare with 500 migrainous patients referred to the same clinic (Lance and Anthony, 1966). No significant difference in the family or personal history of epilepsy and allergy could be found between the two groups (Table 10.1). Medina and Diamond (1976), making a similar comparison, could not demonstrate any difference in the incidence of allergy or of IgE (immunoglobulin E) levels between migrainous and control groups. Bille (1962) also found that the incidence of allergy and epilepsy was no higher in migrainous children than in normal controls.

These observations make it clear that there is no primary relationship between migraine, epilepsy or allergy. It does not deny the possibility that allergic disturbances or delayed hypersensitivity may trigger a migraine attack, or that the vasoconstrictive phase of migraine may precipitate epileptic phenomena in patients predisposed by their genetic constitution or a focal cortical lesion.

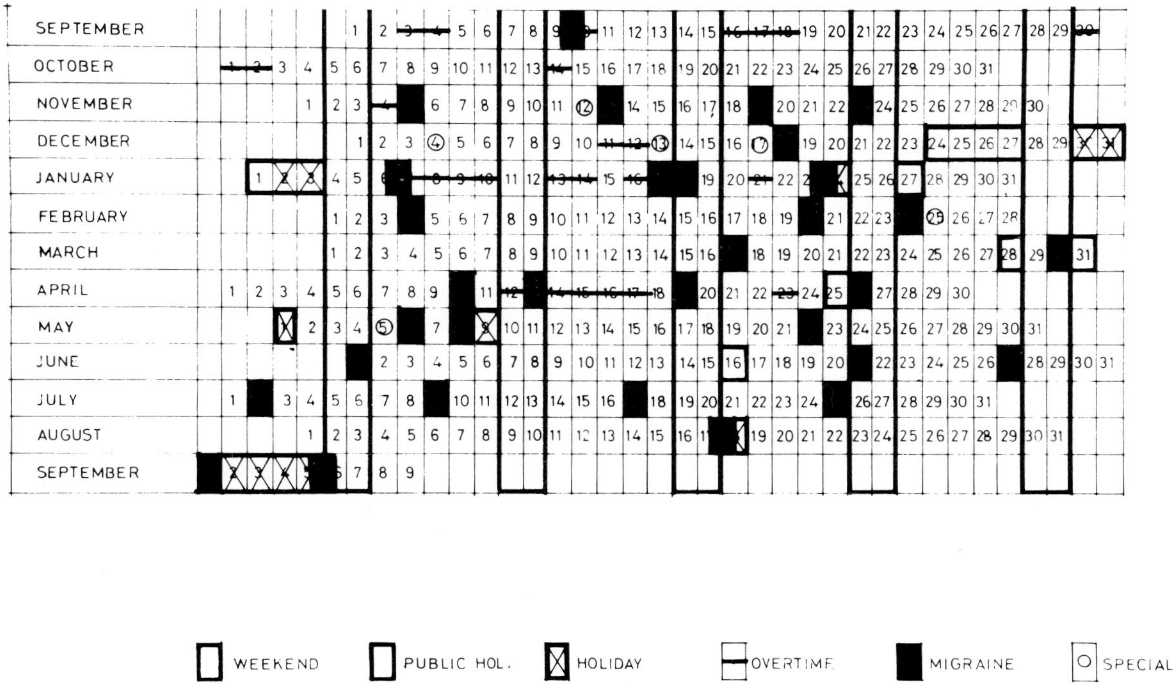

Figure 10.1 Record of headaches and precipitating factors kept by a meticulous migrainous patient

TABLE 10.1
Personal and family history of migraine, epilepsy, allergy and
vomiting attacks in Migraine and Tension Headache

	Personal History			Family History		
	Migraine (per cent)	*Tension (per cent)*	*Significance of difference*	*Migraine (per cent)*	*Tension (per cent)*	*Significance of difference*
Migraine	100.0	0	Not applicable	46·0	18	$P = < 0.001$
Epilepsy	1.6	2	Not significant	2·4	3	Not significant
Allergy	17.4	13	Not significant	8·2	6	Not significant
Childhood vomiting	23.2	12	$P = < 0.02$			

CASE REPORT

The following illustrates a case of temporal lobe epilepsy associated with migraine.

A boy aged 16 years had been subject to 'the thing' about once a week since the age of 8 years. 'The thing' consisted of 'seeing something in my mind like a part of my past life', a sensation which lasted for less than a minute. It could represent some event well remembered or be stylized 'like a cartoon or a picture'. His words were jumbled, he could not read and wrote nonsense while the attack was upon him. About once a month 'the thing' lasted longer than usual, perhaps as long as 15 minutes on occasions, and was followed by nausea and unilateral headache which was nearly always left-sided.

He had been born of an instrumental labour and quivered down the right side shortly after birth. On examination he had a right homonymous hemianopia. Electroencephalography disclosed a left posterior temporal sharp and slow wave focus. An air encephalogram demonstrated a porencephalic cyst which occupied the major part of the posterior quadrant of the left hemisphere. His temporal lobe attacks were controlled by phenytoin and carbamazepine. His migraine headaches responded to sublingual ergotamine tartrate and abated when methysergide was added to the anticonvulsant medication. The history suggests that temporal lobe epilepsy was initiated by the prodromal vasoconstrictive phase of migraine on some occasions bur recurred independently at other times.

In the survey (Lance and Anthony, 1971) mentioned above, a past history of vomiting attacks in childhood was found significantly more frequently in migrainous patients (23 per cent) than patients with muscle-contraction headache (12 per cent), thus supporting the view that cyclical vomiting of childhood may be a precursor of adult migraine. Most children will admit to some sort of headache at the time of their vomiting attacks. Abdominal pain may accompany vomiting attacks of childhood, but cannot be regarded as a migraine equivalent if the only symptom is recurrent abdominal pain. In other words, abdominal symptoms are common in migraine, but it is doubtful whether such an entity as 'abdominal migraine' exists.

Site of headache

Migraine headache is chiefly unilateral in two-thirds of patients and bilateral in the other third (Lance and Anthony, 1971). In about one-fifth of patients, the pain habitually affects the same side of the head in each attack (Selby and Lance, 1960). The pain may be felt deeply behind the eye, but more commonly involves the frontal and temporal regions. It may extend over the entire head and radiate down to the face, or even to the neck and shoulders. In other patients it starts as a dull ache in the upper neck and occipital region and radiates forwards. In some patients it may remain limited to the vascular territory of frontal, temporal or occipital arteries.

Quality of headache

Migraine commonly starts as a dull headache which rapidly becomes more severe and assumes a throbbing or pulsating quality which it may lose as the headache continues or intensifies.

Frequency of attacks

Any analysis from a neurological clinic naturally includes patients with more frequent and severe attacks than those encountered in general practice. More than half the patients attending such a clinic experienced between one and four attacks each month (*Figure 10.3*). It is probable

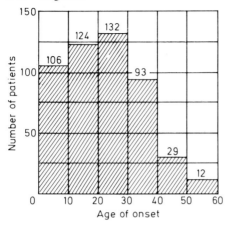

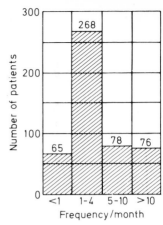

Figure 10.2. The age at which the first migraine attack occurred in 500 patients (from Selby and Lance, 1960). This figure may be compared with that of a different series shown in Figure 9.1. (Reproduced by courtesy of the Editor of the Journal of Neurology, Neurosurgery and Psychiatry)

Figure 10.3. The frequency of migraine attacks in patients attending a neurological clinic (from Selby and Lance, 1960. Reproduced by courtesy of the Editor of the Journal of Neurology, Neurosurgery and Psychiatry)

Figure 10.4. The customary length of each migraine headache reported by 500 patients (from Selby and Lance, 1960. Reproduced by courtesy of the Editor of the Journal of Neurology, Neurosurgery and Psychiatry)

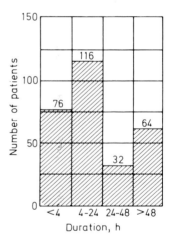

that emotional factors become a great aetiological significance as the frequency of attacks increases. In the 15 per cent of patients who reported more than 10 attacks each month, tension headaches were often present as well and the patients sometimes found it difficult to distinguish between the two (Selby and Lance, 1960). Uncommonly patients may progress to 'status migrainosus' when they awaken each day with recrudescence of their migraine headache.

PLATE I

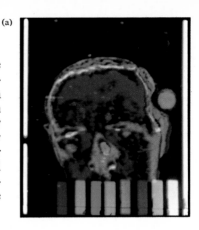
(a)

Facial thermograms in migraine and cluster headache. Each isotherm has been photographed with a different colour filter so that skin temperature may be measured by reference to the colour scale below each photograph. Each colour represents an isotherm separated by 1 degC and the green background or disc represents the reference temperature of 32°C

(a), (b), (c): Changes in migraine headache; (a) before headache, showing symmetry of forehead temperature; (b) at onset of right hemicrania showing that the right side is 1–2 degC cooler than the left; (c) at height of right hemicrania when patient is feeling nauseated. Skin temperature is a little lower but right forehead remains 1 degC cooler than the left

(d), (e): Effect of ergotamine tartrate in migraine headache; (d) patient with right-sided migraine showing that affected side is 1 degC cooler than the left; (e) after oral ergotamine, 3 mg, when headache has subsided, showing restoration of symmetry on forehead

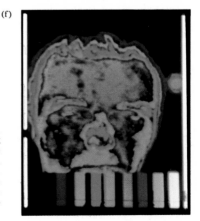
(f)

(f), (g), (h): Changes in cluster headache; (f) before cluster headache, showing symmetry of forehead temperature; (g) early phase of cluster headache with cold patch extending over right eye on painful side; (f) later, when cold patch has disappeared and temple and cheek are warmer on the affected side. (*From Lance and Anthony, 1971*)

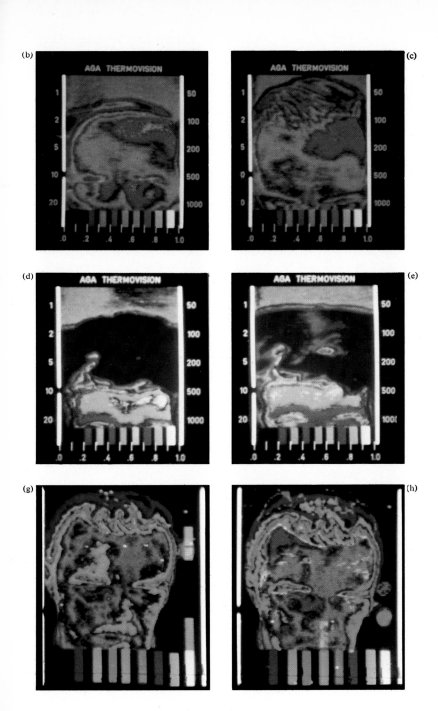

Duration of attacks

The headache persists for less than one day in about two-thirds of patients (*Figure 10.4*), although a feeling of exhaustion and lethargy may remain for several days afterwards.

Time and mode of onset

Migraine headache may start at any time of the day, when it may be preceded by focal neurological symptoms such as visual disturbance. More commonly, the patient awakens in the early morning with the headache already present. Before an attack the patient may experience euphoria or other mood changes, increased appetite and thirst, a craving for sweet things, or drowsiness, all symptoms suggesting a hypothalamic disturbance.

ASSOCIATED PHENOMENA

Vascular changes

The patient with migraine often notices increased pulsation and tenderness of the superficial temporal arteries during a headache, and finds that pressure over the vessel will reduce the intensity of headache. Veins may become prominent over forehead or temple and the conjunctival vessels are usually dilated. The skin may flush, but is more commonly pale and sweating in severe attacks. Hands and feet often feel cold. Patients with migraine may rarely have a fever.

Skin temperature

The temperature of the forehead and scalp may be measured rapidly and conveniently by means of a thermovision camera (*Figure 10.5*). This device incorporates an infrared detector and rapid scanner and displays a picture on a television screen in which the intensity of light is proportional to skin temperature. The AGA thermovision camera is equipped to display separately each isotherm at a selected interval, such as 1 deg C, and each isotherm may be photographed with a different colour filter so that the resulting picture displays the superimposed isotherms like a contour map (Plate 1). Using this device,

Lance and Anthony (1971) studied 15 control subjects, 10 migrainous subjects and 5 patients with cluster headache. Their experience was enlarged by study of another 100 normal subjects in a survey of cerebral vascular disease. Of the 115 normal individuals, 7 showed an asymmetrical facial thermogram. Four of these were rescreened and were then found to be normal. In contrast to this, 8 out of the 15 patients with vascular headache showed an asymmetry when free of headache, and 12 out of 15 were abnormal during a headache. Of 13

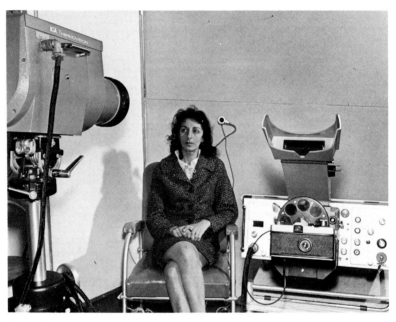

Figure 10.5. Measurement of skin temperature by the AGA thermovision camera. A temperature reference disc can be seen to the left of the patient's head. The camera is seen on the left and the viewing screen on the right

migraine headaches studied, the affected side was cooler by approximately 1 degC in 8 (Plate 1, b, c), was slightly warmer in 2, while the forehead remained symmetrical in 3. When a headache was eased by ergotamine tartrate, the temperature of the forehead became symmetrical (Plate 1, g, h). This supports the suggestion that blood is shunted away from the skin in migraine headache in spite of the dilatation of large scalp arteries.

Sodium and fluid retention

Increase in weight, with or without signs of generalized oedema, is noted by about one-half of migrainous patients before the migraine attack. Oliguria is common before the attack and roughly 30 per cent of patients notice polyuria as the headache subsides. The blood sodium level has been shown to increase before and during headache while serum protein concentration falls (Campbell, Hay and Tonks, 1951). The urinary output of sodium by migrainous subjects between attacks after being given a water load of 1 000 to 1 500 ml is almost double that of controls. There is thus evidence that sodium and fluid retention is associated with migraine, but it is unlikely to be a cause of migraine, since the administration of diuretics, which minimizes weight fluctuations, does not prevent the regular recurrence of migraine headache. Stanford and Greene (1970) suggested that aldosterone might be responsible for the sodium and fluid retention of migraine, and reported the cure of premenstrual migraine by the surgical treatment of Conn's syndrome.

Gastrointestinal disturbance

About 90 per cent of patients feel nauseated with their migraine headache and the majority vomit as well. The passage of one or more loose stools at this phase of the migraine attack is noted by about 20 per cent of patients (Lance and Anthony, 1971). These gastrointestinal symptoms are probably not a reaction to the pain of migraine since they may occur with comparatively mild headaches, particularly in children. It is unlikely that they are caused by intracranial vasoconstriction affecting medullary centres because they are not necessarily associated with vertigo or other symptoms of brainstem ischaemia. Changes in plasma serotonin, described in Chapter 11, might possibly be linked with alteration of gastrointestinal motility.

Photophobia

Some 80 per cent of patients find light unpleasant during migraine headache and prefer to lie down in a darkened room. Photophobia occurs independently of conjunctival vasodilatation and may be a referred pain from irritation of the ophthalmic division of the fifth nerve. Alternatively, it may be just one manifestation of hyperactivity of the special senses, since dislike of noise and strong odours are also common complaints.

Hyperaesthesia

About two-thirds of patients comment on undue sensitivity of the scalp during and after a migraine headache (Selby and Lance, 1960).

FOCAL NEUROLOGICAL SYMPTOMS AND SIGNS

One of the characteristics of migraine which separates it clearly from cluster headache and, of course, from muscle-contraction headache, is its association with transient disturbance of cerebral function in about two-thirds of patients. Visual hallucinations or scotomas are most frequent, occurring in about one-third of all migrainous patients. Fortification spectra are experienced by about 10 per cent of patients, and were given this name because the zig-zag appearance of the hallucination resembles the plan of a fortified town viewed from above. The equivalent term 'teichopsia' is derived from the Greek 'teichos', meaning a wall. Another 25 per cent of patients describe unformed flashes of light ('photopsia') which are white or coloured. Symptoms which originate in areas of cortex other than the occipital lobe are much less common. Paraesthesiae around the mouth and tongue and in both hands may arise from the cortex or from the long sensory tracts in the brainstem. Strictly unilateral paraesthesiae associated with hemiparesis or dysphasia, which is clearly of cortical origin, is encountered in about 4 per cent of patients (Lance and Anthony, 1971). Transient temporal or parietal lobe syndromes may be part of a migraine attack. The author remembers one patient describing the distorted perception of her body image. 'My fingers felt as long as telegraph poles and my mouth with the teeth in it seemed like a cave full of tombstones.' Lewis Carroll suffered from migraine and it has been suggested that some of the inspiration for illusions of vision and body image in *Alice in Wonderland* may have had its origin in migrainous vasospasm. The appeal of the story is little diminished by the knowledge that *Alice in Wonderland* was written before Carroll started to suffer from migraine.

Symptoms arising from the brainstem such as diplopia, vertigo, inco-ordination, ataxia and dysarthia are the only neurological components of the attack in about 25 per cent of patients (Lance and Anthony, 1971). Bickerstaff (1961 a,b) pointed out that severe brainstem symptoms in migraine were often associated with faintness, fainting or sudden loss of consciousness. He attributed this to constriction of the basilar artery which supplies the midbrain reticular formation responsible for the maintenance of consciousness. This is borne out by the experience of the author's clinic, since 7 per cent of patients with symptoms referable to the vertebrobasilar arterial system had fainted on occasions during their attacks, whereas none of those with cortical symptoms arising from areas supplied by the carotid artery had done so (Lance and Anthony, 1971). On the other hand, confusional states without loss of consciousness were more common in the latter group. At times behaviour may be quite bizarre at the height of a migraine headache, such as that of a woman who left her young child in the bath and ran aimlessly down her suburban street.

A confusional state lasting up to several hours is not uncommon as a presenting feature in juvenile migraine (Gascon and Barlow, 1970). A more prolonged stuporous or comatose state lasting for up to 7 days has also been described. The author has encountered migraine stupor in patients aged from 10 to 52 years (Lee and Lance, 1977). Most were associated with homonymous hemianopia, ataxia, inco-ordination and dysarthria while some had a dilated pupil on one side, all suggesting a disturbance of the vertebrobasilar arterial system and its posterior cerebral continuation. Confused, aggressive and hysterical behaviour was noted at some stages of the illness in most patients which led to the diagnosis of hysteria being considered.

The wide variety of migrainous symptoms cannot be covered adequately in a book of this size and the reader is referred to monographs by Klee (1968), Pearce (1969), Sacks (1970) and Wolff (1972) for further details. When focal neurological symptoms and signs outlast the usual duration of migraine headache, the condition is known as complicated migraine.

Complicated migraine

Permanent damage to the central nervous system and the retina may be caused by migraine. The most common defects are a partial or complete homonymous hemianopia and retinal defects (Carroll, 1970) but hemiparesis, hemianaesthesia and other cerebral or brainstem disturbances have been described. Abnormalities of the vestibular system (Raffaelli and Menon, 1975) may also fall into this category Monocular visual loss after migraine is usually caused by retinal vascular occlusion, central serous retinopathy or, rarely, by retinal or vitreous haemorrhages. A case of ischaemic papillopathy has been reported (McDonald and Sanders, 1971). The introduction of computerized tomography has enabled the visualization of cerebral infarction, cerebral oedema and areas of cortical atrophy in migrainous patients, indicating that migraine is not always a benign disorder (Cala and

Mastaglia, 1976; Hungerford, du Boulay and Zilkha, 1976; Mathew *et al.*, 1977).

PRECIPITATING FACTORS

It is possible that anyone may suffer a migraine headache given sufficient stimulus and that the migraine sufferer has a lower threshold to various stimuli than his or her headache-free counterparts. Normal persons have experienced migrainous phenomena for the first time when subjected to rapid changes in barometric pressure in compression or decompression chambers (Anderson *et al.*, 1965; Engel, Ferris and Romano, 1945) or when given an infusion of prostaglandin E_1, (Carlson, Ekelund and Orö, 1968). The threshold for migraine appears to be a familial characteristic although not bound by any consistent hereditary pattern. The effectiveness of trigger factors appears to depend upon the rapidity of change in the internal or external environment.

Trauma

Some precipitating factors act rapidly. Matthews (1972) has reported that soccer players who 'head' the ball may experience blurring of vision within minutes, followed by migraine headache. Haas and his colleagues (1975) described migrainous symptoms, numbness and weakness of one side of the body and speech difficulties, starting 20 minutes or so after mild head injuries in children. These symptoms were followed in most patients by a typical headache and nausea. In their experience, precipitation of migraine by trauma tended to run in families. Presumably in this instance jarring of cranial vessels initiates the migrainous process by causing vasospasm.

Stress

Stress is probably the most commonly recognized precipitant of migraine (Henryk-Gutt and Rees, 1973). A number of the author's patients have described the onset of classic migraine within minutes of an emotional shock, in which case the mechanism may involve the autonomic nervous system and the release of humoral agents. Noise, glare, flickering light or unpleasant weather conditions can induce nervous tension and evoke an attack of migraine.

Relaxation after stress, particularly if this is accompanied by sleeping late in the mornings, may initiate migraine, the so-called 'weekend headache'. Presumably the cranial vessels have been maintained in a state of tonic vasoconstriction during the pressures of the working week, and the sudden lowering of emotional tone (and of the circulating agents which regulate vasoconstriction) may permit unrestrained vasodilatation and the headache which follows.

Sleep

Migraine headache not uncommonly awakens a patient from sleep. Dexter and Riley (1975) have shown that the onset of headache was related to lightening of sleep, the onset of the rapid eye movement (REM) phase, in 11 of 19 instances. The blood serotonin level falls at this time and there are changes in catecholamine levels which will be discussed in the next chapter.

Weather

The effect of sudden changes in barometric pressure in triggering a migraine attack have already been mentioned. Many patients believe that changes in the weather, particularly thunderstorms, may be responsible for migraine. Sulman and his colleagues (1970) have studied the effects of a hot dry wind, known as the Shirav, in Israel. They point out that hot winds are notorious for causing irritability and headache. They list the Santa Ana of Southern California, Arizona desert winds, the Argentine Zonda, the Sirocco of the Mediterranean, the Maltese Xlokk, the Chamsin of Arab countries, the Foehn of Switzerland, southern Germany and Austria, and the North winds of Melbourne. They attribute the symptoms of nervous tension and headache to increased ionization of the air which may precede the arrival of the hot dry wind, and correlated this with excessive urinary excretion of serotonin.

Food and eating habits

Missing a meal may sometimes precipitate migraine, possibly because of hypoglycaemia which in turn stimulates the production of noradrenaline and other changes discussed in Chapter 11.

About 25 per cent of patients consider that their attacks are provoked by eating certain foods, particularly fatty foods, chocolates and oranges (Selby and Lance, 1960). Tomatoes, onions and pineapples are occasionally mentioned. There is some doubt whether this is a delayed hypersensitivity reaction to the chemical content of these foods, or whether it depends on a conditioned reflex. Wolff (1972) quotes experiments in which incriminated foods were ingested by patients without their knowledge and without a headache ensuing. On the other hand, the giving of capsules containing an inert substance with the suggestion that they contained chocolate or other offending food was often followed by an episode of migraine.

Attention has recently focused on the tyramine content of ripe cheeses and the phenylethylamine content of chocolate. Hanington, Horn and Wilkinson (1970) gave capsules of tyramine, 125 mg, or lactose, 125 mg, to 35 patients who gave a history of their headaches being precipitated by certain foods. The administration of tyramine provoked a headache within 24 hours in 65 out of 83 occasions whereas a headache followed lactose on only 3 out of 48 occasions. This effect could not be confirmed by Moffett, Swash and Scott (1972) who studied 8 patients with 'dietary migraine'. Headache followed the ingestion of tyramine in 5 out of 8 cases and also followed the taking of lactose in 5 out of 8 cases. Sandler *et al.* (1970) found that 4 tyramine-sensitive patients excreted significantly higher levels of the breakdown products of noradrenaline than 4 control subjects after the administration of tyramine. They concluded that sufficient tyramine entered the circulation to bring about noradrenaline release. The urinary excretion of tyramine, free or conjugated, was less in tyramine-sensitive patients than controls on a normal diet or after 100 mg of tyramine orally (Smith, Kellow and Hanington, 1970). It remains uncertain as to whether abnormalities of tyramine metabolism play any part in the genesis of migraine.

Sandler, Youdim and Hanington (1974) reported that chocolate contains phenylethylamine (at least 3 mg in a 2-ounce bar). They found that half of 36 'chocolate-sensitive' subjects developed headache 12 hours after ingestion of phenylethylamine whereas only 6 of them experienced headache after lactose. Recently Moffett, Swash and Scott (1974) compared the effect of eating chocolate with the effect of matched placebo mixtures which contained no derivates of cocoa. The texture and taste of the real chocolate was concealed by additives. Of the 25 patients, all of whom considered that chocolate precipitated their migraine attacks, 8 responded with a headache to chocolate, 5 to placebo, 1 to both and 11 to neither. In a second trial involving 15 of these patients, 5 had a headache after chocolate, 3 after placebo, 1 after both and 5 after neither. It is of interest that one patient of mine claims that the only thing which will *prevent* her migraine developing is to eat dark chocolate and keeps a quarter-pound block in the glovebox of her car for this purpose.

Hormonal changes

Johannis van der Linden in *De Hemicrania Menstrua* (1666) described a unilateral headache accompanied by nausea and vomiting, recurring in the Marchioness of Brandenburg each month 'during the menstrual flux'.

The periodicity of migraine is related to the menstrual cycle in about 60 per cent of women patients, the headaches appearing just before, during or after the menses. Migraine is relieved by pregnancy in about 60 per cent of women, but this does not depend upon a previous association with menstruation, although there is a positive correlation. Of women whose migraine was linked with the menses, 64 per cent lost their headache during pregnancy, compared with 48 per cent of those in whom this relationship was absent (Lance and Anthony, 1966). There is no link-up between relief during pregnancy and the sex of the foetus. On the other hand, some patients may experience migraine for the first time during pregnancy.

Somerville (1972b) undertook a similar survey of 200 women attending an antenatal clinic during the last 4 weeks of pregnancy. He found that 31 patients had been subject to migraine headache in the 12 months before becoming pregnant, giving an incidence of 15 per cent for women in the reproductive years. Of the 31 patients, 24 improved during pregnancy, 7 becoming completely free of headache. Only 7 patients had developed migraine for the first time in the current pregnancy, mostly in the first trimester. Somerville found that there was no significant difference in the plasma progesterone of those women whose migraine has improved 98.4 ng/ml, those women whose migraine continued during pregnancy (101.2 ng/ml) and the non-migrainous control patients (119.4 ng/ml).

Somerville (1971, 1972b) has clarified the relationship of migraine to the hormonal changes of the menstrual cycle. Normal and migrainous women were found to have a similar fluctuation of hormonal levels. Plasma oestradiol rose to an early pre-ovulatory peak, followed by a rapid fall, then a secondary rise during the luteal phase with a final fall before menstruation (*Figure 10.6*). Plasma progesterone remained low during menstruation and the follicular phase, then increased at or just after mid-cycle to a plateau during the luteal phase, then declined premenstrually. There was no significant difference between the peak progesterone concentrations in migrainous and non-migrainous women.

Premenstrual migraine occurred regularly during or after plasma oestradiol and progesterone fell to their lowest levels. To determine which of these hormones was the more influential in triggering migraine headache, Somerville treated 6 women with progesterone and 6 women with oestradiol in the premenstrual phase while measuring their hormonal levels daily. He found that the administration of progesterone

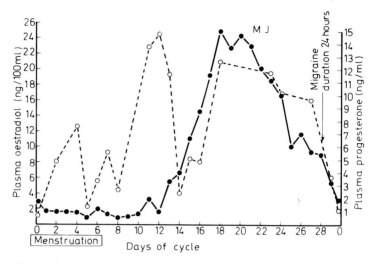

Figure 10.6. Plasma oestradiol (interrupted line) and plasma progesterone (continuous line) estimated daily during a normal menstrual cycle. Premenstrual migraine occurs during the falling phase of both curves (from Somerville, 1972a, by courtesy of the editor of 'Neurology'.)

to maintain artificially high blood levels postponed uterine bleeding, but that the migraine attack occurred in 5 of the 6 women at the anticipated time in the cycle (*Figure 10.7*). On the other hand, the injection of oestradiol did not postpone menstruation but delayed the onset of migraine headache in all patients by 3 to 9 days (*Figure 10.8*). Migraine began after the oestradiol level fell below 20 ng/100 ml and could not be postponed further if another injection of oestradiol was given at this time. Two other women had consistently low levels of progesterone indicating the absence of ovulation. One developed migraine 10 days after an injection of oestradiol, followed on the eleventh day by oestrogen-withdrawal bleeding. The second patient, who was menopausal, suffered a typical episode of migraine as the oestrogen level fell 9 days after injection, without any withdrawal bleeding.

It is therefore apparent that the withdrawal of oestrogen, rather than progesterone, sets in motion a series of changes which culminate in the onset of migraine. This could account for the mid-cycle headache which afflicts some women in addition to menstrual migraine. There is

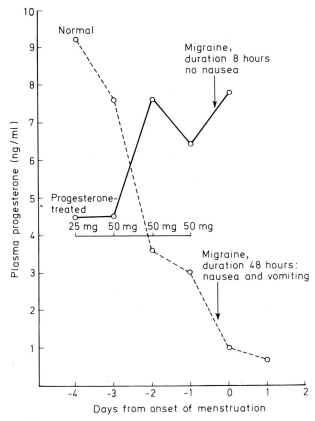

Figure 10.7. Progesterone-treated cycle (continuous line) and normal cycle (interrupted line) in the same patient. Migraine occurs at the usual time in spite of high blood levels of progesterone (from Somerville, 1971, by courtesy of the editor of 'Neurology')

probably some intermediary between oestrogen withdrawal and the sequelae of menstruation and migraine. The prostaglandins are possible contenders because of their actions on the uterus, and the known effect of PGE_1 in precipitating migraine when infused into normal subjects (Carlson, Ekelund and Orö, 1968).

The use of oral contraceptive tablets commonly exacerbates migraine (Whitty, Hockaday and Whitty, 1966). Dalton (1975) found that 34 per cent of women taking contraceptive pills and 60 per cent of those who had ceased to take them considered that their migraine was worse while on the pill. Permanent neurological deficit has been

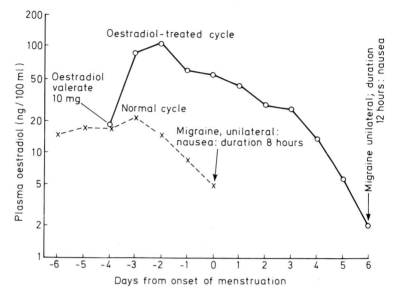

Figure 10.8. Oestrogen-treated cycle (continuous line) and normal cycle (interrupted line) in the same patient. The onset of migraine is postponed until the oestrogen level falls (from Somerville, 1972b, by courtesy of the editor of 'Neurology')

reported in patients whose phase of intracranial vasoconstriction was prolonged while taking oral contraceptives (Gardner, Van den Noort and Horenstein, 1967).

Vasodilatation

Alcohol and other vasodilators are well recognized as inducers of migraine or cluster headache and vasoconstrictor drugs are instrumental in ending it.

Exertion may provoke a migraine attack or other varieties of vascular headache. Pressure over dilated scalp arteries or the application of cold packs will often relieve the headache. The reason for hot packs relieving some patients' attacks is less obvious but could be that capillary vasodilatation reduces the internal pressure and hence the distension of larger proximal vessels.

Associated diseases

Migraine may be aggravated by hypertension (Walker, 1959) and aldosteronism (Stanford and Greene, 1970). It has been reported as a symptom of hyper-pre-beta lipoproteinaemia, possibly because of changes in plasma viscosity or red cell aggregation, and it disappears with restoration of serum lipids to normal (Leviton and Camenga, 1969). There is still some dispute as to the significance of cervical spondylosis and whether compression of the vertebral arteries or their sympathetic plexus by osteophytes can give rise to 'migraine cervicale'.

PHYSICAL EXAMINATION

There are no physical signs of migraine detectable between attacks. Hearing a bruit over the skull or orbits may give rise to concern and warrant carotid angiography to exclude the presence of an intracranial aneurysm or angioma. In one series of 500 patients, 10 were found to have an audible cranial bruit (Selby and Lance, 1960). Two were children under the age of 10 years in whom skull bruits are usually not of any significance. In 4 adult patients the bruit was heard over both eyes, and in 4 it was unilateral. Carotid angiograms in 3 of the latter were completely normal.

In the above-mentioned series, a blood pressure of more than 150 mm systolic and 100 mm diastolic was found in 13 per cent of patients. Hypertension is said to be significantly more common over the age of 50 years in migrainous patients than in the general population and this is discussed in Chapter 7.

While a migraine headache is in progress, excessive pulsation of temporal arteries may be noted and veins are often prominent on forehead and temple. The face and scalp are commonly pale and sweaty in severe attacks. The patient may be mentally confused, stuporous or even lose consciousness for a brief time. Speech may be slurred (dysarthria) or there may be inability to choose the correct word or phrase (dysphasia). There may be a transient Horner's syndrome or paresis of the third cranial nerve. More rarely, hemiparesis or involuntary movements may be observed at the height of the attack. The patient may be ataxic and have difficulty with co-ordination. Such patients of mine have been suspected of drunkenness and questioned by the police when struggling to get home after being taken unawares by a migraine attack. They now carry a letter explaining the vagaries of migraine.

REFERENCES

Anderson, B., Jr, Heyman, A., Whalen, R.E. and Saltzman, H.A. (1965). Migraine-like phenomena after decompression from hyperbaric environment. *Neurology* 15, 1035

Bickerstaff, E.R. (1961a). Basilar artery migraine *Lancet* 1, 15

Bickerstaff, E.R. (1961b). Impairment of consciousness in migraine. *Lancet* 2, 1057

Bickerstaff, E.R. (1964). Ophthalmoplegic migraine. *Revue Neurol.* 110, 582

Bille, B. (1962). Migraine in school-children. *Acta paediat. Stockh.,* 51, (Suppl. 136) 1

Bradshaw, P. and Parsons, M. (1965). Hemiplegic migraine; a clinical study. *Q. J. Med.* 34, 65

Brewis, M., Poskanzer, D.C., Rolland, C. and Miller, H. (1966). Neurological disease in an English city. *Acta neurol. scand.* 42, Suppl. 24

Cala, L.A., and Mastaglia, F.L. (1976). Computerised axial tomography findings in patients with migrainous headaches. *Br. med. J.* 2, 149

Campbell, D.A., Hay, K.M., and Tonks, E.M. (1951). An investigation of salt and water balance in migraine. *Br. med. J.* 2, 1424

Carlson, L.A., Ekelund, L-G and Orö, L. (1968). Clinical and metabolic effects of different doses of prostaglandin E in man. *Acta med. scand.* 183, 423

Carroll, J.D. (1970). Complicated migraine. In *Kliniske aspekter i Migraene-forskningen,* p. 88. Copenhagen: Nordlundes Bogtrykkeri

Dalsgaard-Nielsen, J. (1970). Some aspects of the epidemiology of migraine in Denmark. In *Kliniske Aspekter i migraeneforskningen,* p. 18. Copenhagen: Nordlundes Bogtrykkeri.

Dalton, K. (1975). Migraine and oral contraceptives. *Headache* 15, 247

Dexter, J.D. and Riley, T.L. (1975). Studies in nocturnal migraine. *Headache* 15, 51

Engel, G.L., Ferris, E.B. and Romano, J. (1945). Focal electroencephalographic changes during the scotomas of migraine. *Am. J. med. Sci.* 209, 650

Gardner, J.H., Van den Noort, S. and Horenstein, S. (1967). Cerebrovascular disease in young women taking oral contraceptives. *Neurology, Minneap.* 17, 297

Gascon, G. and Barlow, C. (1970). Juvenile migraine presenting as an acute confusional state. *Pediatrics* 45, 628

Gowers, W.R. (1893). *A Manual of Diseases of the Nervous System.* Vol. 2. p.838 Philadelphia: Blakiston

Haas, D.C., Pineda, G.S. and Lourie, H. (1975). Juvenile head trauma syndromes and their relationship to migraine. *Archs. Neurol.* 32, 727

Hanington, E., Horn, M. and Wilkinson, M. (1970). Further observations on the effects of tyramine. In *Background to Migraine.* Third British Migraine Symposium, p. 120. London: Heinemann.

Henryk-Gutt, R. and Rees, W.L. (1973). Psychological aspects of migraine. *J. psychosom. Res.* 17, 141

Herberg, L.J. (1975). The hypothalamus and aminergic pathways in migraine. In *Modern Topics in Migraine*, Ed. J. Pearce, p. 85. London; Heinemann

Hungerford, G.D., du Boulay, G.H., and Zilkha, K.J. (1976). Computerized axial tomography in patients with severe migraine: a preliminary report. *J. Neurol. Psychiat.* **39**, 990

Klee, A. (1968). *A Clinical Study of Migraine with Particular Reference to the Most Severe Cases.* p. 190. Copenhagen: Munksgaard

Lance, J.W. and Anthony, M. (1966). Some clinical aspects of migraine. *Archs. Neurol.* **15**, 356

Lance, J.W. and Anthony, M. (1971). Thermographic studies in vascular headache. *Med. J. Aust.* **1**, 240

Lee, C.H. and Lance, J.W. (1977). Migraine stupor. *Headache* **17**, 32

Leviton, A. and Camenga, D. (1969). Migraine associated with hyper-pre-beta-lipoproteinaemia. *Neurology* **19**, 963

Mathew, N.T., Meyer, J.S., Welch, K.M.A., and Neblett, C.R. (1977). Abnormal CT scans in migraine. *Headache* **16**, 272

Matthews, W.B. (1972). Footballer's migraine. *Br. med. J.,* **1**, 326

McDonald, W.I. and Sanders, M.D. (1971). Migraine complicated by ischaemic papillopathy. *Lancet* **3**, 521

Medina, J.L. and Diamond, S. (1976). Migraine and atopy. *Headache* **15**, 271

Moffett, A., Swash, M. and Scott, D.F. (1972). Effect of tyramine in migraine: a double-blind study. *J. Neurol. Neurosurg. Psychiat.* **35**, 496

Moffett, A.M., Swash, M. and Scott, D.F. (1974). Effect of chocolate in migraine: a double-blind study. *J. Neurol. Neurosurg. Psychiat.* **37**, 445

Pearce, J. (1969). *Migraine, Clinical Features, Mechanisms and Management.* Springfield: Thomas

Raffaelli, E. Jr and Menon, A.D. (1975). Migraine and the limbic system. *Headache* **15**, 69

Sacks, O.W. (1970). *Migraine. Evolution of a Common Disorder.* London: Faber and Faber

Sandler, M. Youdim, M.B.H. and Hanington, E. (1974). A phenylethylamine oxidasing defect in migraine. *Nature* **250**, 335

Sandler, M., Youdim, M.B.H., Southgate, J. and Hanington, E. (1970). The role of tyramine in migraine: some possible biochemical mechanisms. In *Background to Migraine*, Third British Migraine Symposium p. 103. London: Heinemann

Selby, G. and Lance, J.W. (1960). Observations on 500 cases of migraine and allied vascular headache. *J. Neurol. Neurosurg. Psychiat.* **23**, 23

Smith, I., Kellow, A.H. and Hanington, E. (1970). Tyramine metabolism in dietary migraine. In *Background to Migraine*, Third British Migraine Symposium p. 120. London: Heinemann

Somerville, B.W. (1971). The role of progesterone in menstrual migraine. *Neurology, Minneap.* **21**, 853

Somerville, B.W. (1972a). The role of estradiol withdrawal in the etiology of menstrual migraine. *Neurology, Minneap.* **22**, 355

Somerville, B.W. (1972b). A study of migraine in pregnancy. *Neurology, Minneap.* **22**, 824

Stanford, E. and Greene, R. (1970). A case of migraine cured by treatment of Conn's syndrome. In *Background to Migraine* Third British Migraine Symposium p. 53. London: Heinemann.

Sulman, F.G., Danon, A., Pfeifer, Y., Tal, E. and Weller, C.P. (1970). Urinalysis of patients suffering from climatic heat stress. *Int. J. Biomet.* **14**, 205

Sweetnam, M.T. (1961). An enquiry into the treatment of migraine. *J. Coll. gen. Practnrs Res. Newsl.* **4**, 538

Walker, C.H. (1959). Migraine and its relationship to hypertension. *Br. med. J.* **2**, 1430

Waters, W.E. (1975). Epidemiology. In *Modern Topics in Migraine* Ed. J. Pearce. p. 8. London: Heinemann

Waters, W.E. and O'Connor, P.J. (1970). The clinical validation of a headache questionnaire. In *Background to Migraine,* Third British Migraine Symposium. p. 1. London: Heinemann

Whitty, C.W.M. (1953). Familial hemiplegic migraine. *J. Neurol. Neurosurg. Psychiat.* **16**, 172

Whitty, C.W.M. and Hockaday, J.M. (1968). Migraine. A follow-up study of 92 patients. *Br. med. J.* **1**, 735

Whitty, C.W.M., Hockaday, J.M. and Whitty, M.M. (1966). The effect of oral contraceptives on migraine. *Lancet* **1**, 856

Wolff, H.G. (1972). Headache and other head pain. (Third edition, revised by D.J. Dalessio) New York: Oxford University Press

Eleven

The Pathogenesis
of Migraine

*Headache, which is one of the most serious complaints, is sometimes
occasioned by an intemperament solely; sometimes by a redundance of
humours, and sometimes by both . . .*

Paul of Aegina, circa A.D. 600
(Adams, 1844)

THE MECHANISM OF PAIN PRODUCTION IN
MIGRAINE HEADACHE

The pain of migraine was long suspected to be of vascular origin
because of the observation that arteries and veins were prominent in
the forehead and temples during the attack and that pressure over the
scalp vessels or the common carotid artery in the neck eased the pain to
some extent. In 1938, Graham and Wolff published an important paper
showing that the amplitude of pulsation of scalp arteries increased with
the onset of migraine and correlated well with the severity of the headache at each stage of the attack. The injection of ergotamine tartrate
reduced the pulsation of the extracranial arteries by 50 per cent at the
same time as the headache was relieved. Graham and Wolff recorded
the pulsation of the CSF as an indirect method of measuring dilatation
of intracranial vessels and found that there was no increase during
migraine headache or any significant reduction after the injection of
ergotamine tartrate. Irrespective of their contribution to headache,
the intracranial vessels are thought to dilate in some migraine attacks.
On one occasion a burr-hole exploration was done at the height of a
migraine headache and a tight, non-pulsating dura was found. The

brain looked oedematous and cerebral blood vessels were seen to be dilated (Goltman, 1935/36).

Further evidence about the vascular nature of migraine, although not discriminating between the part played by intracranial and extra-cranial arteries, was brought forward by Wolff (1972), who spun patients in a human centrifuge at a positive acceleration of 2·0 g with a complete relief of headache. It is a pity that this treatment is impractical as an office procedure.

Thus the evidence has slowly accumulated that migraine is of vascular origin and that it is chiefly the extracranial arteries which are at fault. Artificial distension of one superficial temporal artery will reproduce the pain of migraine in the temple (Wolff, 1972). It has been shown that the pulsation of the superficial temporal artery is larger than normal in migrainous subjects, even at times of freedom from headache, and that it becomes more variable 3 to 4 days before a headache (Tunis and Wolff, 1953). Just before an attack, while a patient is experiencing the phase of visual scotomas, the amplitude of pulsation is at its lowest. As the headache develops, the pulsation increased on the affected side (Tunis and Wolff, 1952). Conjunctival vessels may dilate on the side of headache and become less sensitive to the local application of vasoconstrictor agents such as noradrenaline (Ostfeld and Wolff, 1955). Blau and Davis (1970) have recently reported that the conjunctival vessels constricted in half the patients observed and dilated in the remainder. The changes were bilateral although more evident on the side of headache, and intravascular red cell aggregation was seen in all cases. Tissue clearance studies using radioactive sodium have shown that skin blood flow increases in the frontotemporal region during migraine, more so on the side of the headache (Elkind, Friedman and Grossman, 1964).

These observations make it clear that the scalp arteries dilate and cause headache in migraine. How can this be so, when no normal person experiences headache after strenuous exercise or a hot shower or bath which causes obvious dilatation of scalp vessels? One explanation is that dilatation of the capillaries does not keep pace with the arteries in migraine, so that the vessel wall becomes overdistended. There is an analogous situation when cold is applied to the forehead of normal persons. The small vessels constrict in response to cold while the large vessels are still dilated; the subject feels pain at this stage, although the pain is not really the same as that of migraine. This concept of imbalance between the calibre of large and small vessels is supported by the appearance of most patients who look pale during migraine headache in spite of their bounding temporal pulses. Skin temperature is lower on the affected side of the head in the majority of migrainous patients (Plate 1). Lund (1957) has claimed that the administration of substances which dilate small vessels relieves migraine headache and restores the shape of the arterial pulse wave to normal, even though the amplitude remains constant at its former high level. It is hard to reconcile this idea with the knowledge that skin blood flow (measured by injected isotopes) is increased during migraine (Elkind, Friedman and Grossman, 1964). Possibly shunting of blood may take place deep to the constricted skin capillaries, thus removing injected isotope rapidly, while an increased pressure is sustained in the major scalp arteries. Heyck (1969) found that the arteriovenous oxygen saturation difference between arterial blood and venous blood from the external jugular vein (mean 4·8 vol. per cent) was normally less than that between arterial blood and the cubital vein (mean 8·75 vol. per cent) but fell to a mean of 1·5 vol. per cent on the side of headache during a migraine attack and to 3·5 vol. per cent on the relatively painless side. After migraine had abated, the value on the previously affected side had returned to 4·15 vol. per cent in the 6 patients studied. This indicates that scalp blood flow is greater than that of the arm relative to its metabolic requirements and suggests that flow is augmented in the scalp during migraine headache, even though the skin capillaries are constricted.

An important factor in the production of pain from migrainous vessels appears to be the accumulation around the dilated arteries of various substances which are capable of sensitizing them to pain. A polypeptide has been found in the periarterial fluid sampled during migraine headache which is similar to the polypeptide found in blister fluid. Wolff and his colleagues called this substance 'neurokinin' and thought that it could be responsible for setting up a sterile inflammatory response in the vessel (Chapman et al., 1960; Ostfeld et al., 1957). They considered that biopsies of the scalp arteries taken at the time of headache showed pallor and homogenous staining of the perivascular tissue which suggested that the vessel wall was oedematous (Ostfeld et al., 1957). These changes are equivocal and recent observers have not agreed that there is any definite abnormality (Adams, Orton and Zilkha, 1968). However, the presence of 'neurokinin' has to be considered in discussing the mechanism of migraine, since it is known to be a potent pain-provoking substance like bradykinin. Sicuteri (1963) has reported that mast cells are reduced in number and in granulation, in biopsy specimens taken at the time of headache. Thonnard-Neumann and Taylor (1968) found that the number of basophil leucocytes in blood taken from an ear-lobe on the side of headache was increased in comparison with the headache-free side, although this may be a non-specific reaction to vasodilatation.

The basophil cells on the affected side were degranulated. (Thonnard-Neumann, 1969). The local release of heparin and histamine from mast and basophil cells may be associated with the accumulation of kinins in the vessel wall and possibly with the local action of serotonin in the production of pain from distended arteries during migraine.

Enough evidence has been brought forward now to make it clear that the control of extracranial blood vessels must be faulty in migraine. Histological studies have shown that the vascular pattern in some other parts of the body is abnormal in migrainous patients. Capillary loops in the nail bed and mucous membrane of the lip are of immature appearance in the majority of migraine patients (Hauptmann, 1946; Redisch and Pelzer, 1943), and unusual groups of arterioles have been found in endometrial biopsies of migrainous women (Grant, 1965). There are no similar observations on the vascular pattern of the scalp which would be of more direct relevance to the problem we are considering.

Sicuteri (1976) has administered parachlorphenylalanine, which inhibits serotonin synthesis, to migrainous patients. He found that the veins of treated patients became more responsive to the effect of serotonin, constricting in response to 5 per cent of their previous threshold dose. Of the 18 patients treated, 4 complained of spontaneous pains in the face, trunk and limbs which led Sicuteri to postulate that central serotonin deficiency in migrainous patients resulted in increased pain perception. He reported that giving L-tryptophan, the precursor of serotonin, to migrainous patients by daily intravenous injection caused improvement in about 50 per cent of patients. There is certainly evidence to implicate serotonin in the mechanism of migraine and it is logical to assume that changes in central synapses which depend on serotonin as a transmitter substance may run parallel with those which have been demonstrated in the blood. Nevertheless, the potent vascular effects of serotonin appear at the moment to be more relevant to the production of pain in migraine than any increased central susceptibility to pain.

THE CAUSE OF FOCAL NEUROLOGICAL
SYMPTOMS IN MIGRAINE

Neurological symptoms are experienced by about 65 per cent of patients, either preceding or during migraine headache. One-third of patients complain of visual disturbance; 4 per cent notice other cortical symptoms such as aphasia and unilateral paraesthesiae; and one-quarter have vertigo, slurred speech or other brainstem symptoms. Such symptoms may appear transiently and inconstantly or may regularly develop over 10 to 30 minutes, suggesting a slow march of inhibition moving over the cerebral cortex.

Goltman (1935/36) had the unusual opportunity of observing a patient with a frontal skull defect while a migraine attack was in progress. The scalp was depressed at the site of the skull defect when the headache began, but filled up as pain spread over the head until there was a bulging, non-pulsatile mass palpable at the height of the headache, which subsided as the headache wore off. This sequence suggests that a phase of cerebral vasoconstriction was followed by vasodilatation and cerebral oedema. The large cerebral arteries do not usually constrict since the majority of angiograms taken during an attack have been completely normal. Cerebral angiography may be normal in spite of the presence of gross neurological deficit in the prodromal phase of migraine, at a time when blood flow is reduced by 50 per cent in the appropriate brain areas (Skinhøj, 1970). Retrograde flow from the carotid arterial system into the basilar artery has been observed in some cases, indicating reduced flow in the vertebrobasilar territory. Constriction of retinal vessels has been described in patients with unilateral impairment of vision as a prodrome of migraine, and such defects may become permanent as the result of thrombosis of the central retinal artery or its branches. Damage to the cerebral hemispheres or brainstem may also result from migraine, presumably as a result of prolonged ischaemia. The prodromal phase of migraine is accompanied by diminished cerebral blood flow which may be global or may comprise areas of low perfusion in regions which correlate with the clinical symptoms (Simard and Paulson, 1973; Skinhøj, 1970, 1973). Autoregulation is lost (Simard and Paulson, 1973). During the headache cerebral blood flow is increased and this increase may persist after the headache has been eased by the injection of ergotamine tartrate (Norris, Hachinski and Cooper, 1975). This supports the view that migrainous headache depends upon the extracranial rather than the intracranial circulation.

The CSF lactate level increases in migraine whether common or classic, reflecting an increase in anaerobic glycolysis as a result of cerebral ischaemia. The mean value rose from 1·54 (± 0·16) to 2·14 (± 0·58) mmol/litre in 10 patients studied by Skinhøj (1973). Welch et al., (1975) found gamma-aminobutyric acid (GABA) in the CSF of 6 patients during migraine headache but not in 14 headache-free controls, 7 of which were subject to migraine and 7 to tension headache. This may be an indication of increased capillary permeability due to hypoxia. A similar interpretation may be placed on the findings of increased cyclic AMP levels in the CSF of 13 patients sampled during or within 48 hours of a migraine attack (Welch *et al.*, 1976). No change in cyclic AMP occurs in the plasma. There seems little doubt that ischaemia of the cortex or brainstem is the source of focal neurological symptoms and signs in migraine.

Local changes have been recorded in the electroencephalogram from the back of the scalp overlying the visual cortex during the prodromal symptoms of migraine, with focal slow waves appearing over the left occipital region when visual hallucinations were noticed in the right half-field and vice versa. Visual evoked potentials are diminished on the appropriate side during the visual aura of classic migraine and may remain depressed between attacks.

Pre-headache scotomas may be induced by the intravenous infusion of the vasoconstrictor agent noradrenaline and can be relieved in some patients by the use of vasodilators such as amyl nitrite or the inhalation of 10 per cent carbon dioxide in air or oxygen which has a potent effect in dilating intracranial arteries (Wolff, 1972).

These observations all imply that vasoconstriction is important in the genesis of neurological symptoms in migraine but there may be other factors as well. Neurophysiologists recognize a curious reaction called 'spreading depression' which takes place in animal brain when it has been damaged by dehydration or hypoxia (Marshall, 1959). Waves of inhibition move slowly over the cerebral cortex, preventing normal activity. Lashley (1941) plotted the expansion of his own visual scotoma in migraine and calculated that the visual cortex was being suppressed by some process advancing at the rate of about 3 mm each minute. This is the same rate of progress as the 'spreading depression' which interferes with cortical recordings in animal experiments (Milner, 1958). Spreading depression is associated with dilatation of the pial arteries and cerebral oedema but may be preceded by a phase of vaso-constriction (Marshall, 1959). It is tempting to postulate that the vasoconstrictor phase of migraine triggers off the ionic changes responsible for 'spreading depression' which thus causes the slow march of neurological symptoms in migraine.

The third nerve may be temporarily paralyzed in some migraine attacks (ophthalmoplegic migraine) and the mechanism is probably different from that of other symptoms and signs. Wolff has suggested that the third nerve may be compressed by dilated arteries as it passes between the posterior cerebral and superior cerebellar arteries, or that oedema of one cerebral hemisphere may be sufficient to force part of the temporal lobe into the tentorial notch, thus stretching the third nerve (Wolff, 1973)

DISORDERED NEUROVASCULAR CONTROL IN MIGRAINE

Symptoms which are primarily of neural origin include mood changes (commonly euphoria preceding an attack and depression afterwards), increased appetite and thirst, a craving for sweet things and drowsiness, suggesting a hypothalamic disturbance. It is probable that vomiting is of neurohumoral origin since nausea may precede any other migrainous symptom. Adrenaline, noradrenaline, dopamine and Dopa were found to have an emetic action in unanaesthetized cats and dogs when given intravenously or intraperitoneally (Cahen, 1974). The effect was enhanced by MAO inhibitors and blocked by chlorpromazine, reserpine and yohimbine, an alpha-adrenergic blocking agent. A similar emetic effect was produced in cats by 5-hydroxytryptophan, and was also decreased by chlorpromazine and reserpine. Amine-induced vomiting may be mediated through the area postrema of the medulla or the hypothalamus.

The vascular changes of migraine include dilatation and increase in pain sensitivity of large intracranial and extracranial arteries with shunting of blood away from the periphery, resulting in focal neurological symptoms (thought to result from cortical or brainstem ischaemia) and pallor of the skin.

Resting blood flow in the hand is higher in migrainous patients than controls, but the percentage fall in flow that resulted when a cold stimulus is applied was found to be less than in normal subjects (Downey and Frewin, 1972). Responses of the hand vessels to the intra-arterial infusion of noradrenaline and tyramine were the same as in normal subjects.

When skin of the trunk or legs is heated, forearm vessels dilate reflexly in normal subjects. Appenzeller and his colleagues (1963) found that this response was reduced or absent in 8 out of 10 migrainous patients, but this has not been confirmed by more recent experiments (French, Lassers and Desai, 1967; Hockaday, Macmillan and Whitty, 1967; Macmillan and Hockaday, 1966). There have been no comparable observations on the reactions of scalp vessels, which is a pity because they are more pertinent to the problem of migraine. When a migrainous patient stands suddenly, the pulsation of scalp arteries diminishes, unlike those of normal subjects, suggesting that there might be some defect in vasomotor control (Wennerholm, 1961). The adventitial collagen around migrainous arteries absorbs noradrenaline more than that of normal subjects when incubated with noradrenaline (Adams, Orton and Zilkha, 1968). This may be a primary change in the adventitia or be a reaction to repeated dilatation of the vessels.

Many early reports on the effect of surgical procedures in migraine are invalidated by doubtful diagnosis and inadequate follow-up. It is clear that cervical sympathectomy does not provide any lasting benefit in migraine (White and Smithwick, 1944) and section of the greater superficial petrosal nerve does not prevent migraine. Ligation of the external carotid artery or the middle meningeal artery, or both, is unreliable in its effects. Removal of the carotid body on the appropriate side cannot be recommended in the treatment of migraine (Lance, Anthony and Gonski, 1967). The only operation which is of predictable benefit is that of section of trigeminal pathways, which gives relief from pain at the expense of permanent facial analgesia (Penfield, 1932; White and Sweet, 1955).

It may be concluded that there is no convincing evidence at present that the neural control of blood vessels is impaired in migraine, that migraine is caused solely by an abnormal neural discharge, or that operation on nerve pathways will prevent migraine.

If the vascular changes of migraine are not caused by abnormal neural discharge, can they be explained by changes in chemical vasomotor regulation? This will be discussed after presentation of the known metabolic disturbances of migraine.

METABOLIC DISTURBANCES

Electrolytes

Retention of sodium and fluid before and during headache was mentioned in Chapter 10.

Ammonia

Of 15 children with migraine accompanied by vomiting and lethargy, investigated by Russell (1973), 9 had high fasting blood ammonia levels of 70 to 120 μg/100 ml (49–96 μmol/l. The normal range is 10 to 45 μg/100 ml or 7 to 31·5 μmol/l. Ammonia and protein loading tests were positive in 8, with peak levels of 130 to 180 μg/100 ml (91–126 μmol/l), correlated in 6 with migrainous symptomatology. Of 7 patients, 3 were heterozygotes for a defect in ornithine transcarbamylase (OTC) which normally catalyses the conversion of carbamyl phosphate and ornithine to citrulline in the Krebs–Henseleit urea cycle. Ammonia may thus be responsible for stupor in some migrainous patients.

Glucose

Migrainous subjects are unduly sensitive to insulin and blood glucose levels are significantly below those of control subjects during a 2-hour insulin hypoglycaemia test. Steroid output in response to insulin and metapyrone indicate that the hypothalamo-pituitary axis is intact (Rao and Pearce, 1971), but the migrainous patient has a diminished hyperglycaemic response 30 minutes after the injection of glucagon, (De Silva, Ron and Pearce, 1974), indicating impairment of mobilization of glucose from the liver.

Free fatty acids (FFA)

FFA increase in the blood in fasting patients who develop migraine more than in those who do not (Hockaday, Williamson and Whitty, 1971). Anthony (1977) has recently shown that FFA were significantly elevated during migraine headache in 23 out of 30 patients. In 5 patients, oleic acid rose by 63 per cent, palmitic and linoleic acids by 39 per cent each, while stearic acid did not change. FFA may act as agents releasing serotonin from platelets.

Other lipids

Migraine has been reported as a symptom of hyper-pre-beta-lipoproteinaemia, which vanishes when serum lipids are restored to normal. The high triglyceride levels in this disorder may affect the circulation by altering blood viscosity, increasing platelet aggregation or potentiating vasoconstrictor agents (McCalden, Bloom and Rosendorff, 1975).

Prostaglandins are long-chain unsaturated fatty acids with effects on the cerebral circulation, E_1 being the most potent dilator and $F_{2\alpha}$ the most potent constrictor. So far, no change in prostaglandin levels have been detected in the plasma of migrainous patients (Anthony, 1976) although the intravenous infusion of PGE_1 into normal subjects may produce a headache indistinguishable from migraine (Carlson, Ekelund and Orö, 1968). Sandler (1972) suggested that tyramine and possibly serotonin could release prostaglandins from the lung into the pulmonary veins and hence into the systemic and cerebral circulations.

Serotonin

Serotonin is carried in the blood almost entirely in the platelets. There is considerable diurnal and individual variation in blood serotonin levels, so that random sampling is meaningless. Once a baseline has been established for each patient, a slight rise in plasma serotonin may be seen at the onset of a migraine attack and then the level falls sharply with the onset of headache (Anthony, Hinterberger and Lance, 1967; Cumings 1971; Curran, Hinterberger and Lance, 1965).

Mean plasma serotonin has been shown to fall from 0·64 to 0·40 $\mu g/10^9$ platelets (from 3·63 to 2·27 $nmol/10^9$ platelets) in 61 patients during migraine headache (Anthony and Lance, 1975). Somerville (1976) has shown that the same drop can be demonstrated in jugular venous blood as well as forearm venous blood but could not find any change in free serotonin levels. In 1968, Anthony, Hinterberger and Lance demonstrated a serotonin-releasing factor in the blood during migraine headache and this has been confirmed by Dvilansky *et al.*, (1976). Its nature is at present unknown but it is of low molecular weight since it passes through a membrane with a minimum pore size of 50 000 mw (Anthony and Lance, 1975). Various free fatty acids and antigen-antibody complexes are being considered as possible liberators of serotonin.

Plasma serotonin tends to increase after vomiting or diarrhoea during the headache but the effect is inconstant. Serotonin levels do not change in cluster headache or when a headache is induced by air encephalography, even when it is quite as severe as that of migraine and gives rise to nausea and vomiting. Other stressful procedures such as arteriography, gastroscopy and bronchoscopy do not alter the serotonin levels (Anthony, Hinterberger and Lance, 1967). It is thus apparent that the fall in plasma serotonin is specific for migraine headache and not a general response to any form of headache, pain or stress.

The main breakdown product of serotonin, 5-hydroxyindoleacetic acid (5HIAA) is excreted in excess in the urine of some patients during migraine headache (Curran, Hinterberger and Lance, 1965; Sicuteri. Testi and Anselmi, 1961). The urinary concentration of 5HIAA also increases, indicating that the changes cannot be explained by the polyuria which frequently accompanies migraine.

The intramuscular injection of reserpine lowers plasma serotonin. At the same time normal subjects experience a dull headache, and the majority of migrainous patients undergo a typical migraine headache. The intravenous injection of serotonin, 2 to 7·5 mg, in spontaneous or reserpine-induced migraine increases plasma serotonin and alleviates the headache (Anthony, Hinterberger and Lance, 1967; Kimball,

Friedman and Vallejo, 1960). It therefore seems likely that serotonin is one of the humoral agents implicated in migraine headache. Serotonin does not pass readily through the blood-brain barrier and its concentration in the cerebrospinal fluid is not altered during migraine headache (Barrie and Jowett, 1967; Southren and Christoff, 1962). Serotonin reduces glomerular filtration rate, probably as a result of renal vasoconstriction and it is possible that this could account for the oliguria which precedes migraine, and the increased urinary excretion of histidine and lysine which has been reported in migraine (Kimball and Goodman, 1966).

Serotonin induces aggregation of platelets to an extent which depends on the availability of uptake sites on the platelets. If uptake sites are already occupied by serotonin molecules, the platelets cannot aggregate. The lower the blood serotonin level, the less the uptake sites are occupied and the greater the degree of platelet aggregation in response to added serotonin (Hilton and Cumings, 1971). Serotonin-induced aggregation of platelets was found to be greater in migrainous patients than controls whether the specimen was taken at the time of headache or not, implying that migrainous platelets are less able to retain serotonin than those of normal subjects (Hilton and Cumings, 1972).

Kalendovsky and Austin (1975) reported that platelet aggregability was more pronounced in patients with complicated migraine (those with persisting focal neurological signs) but Couch and Hassanein (1976) found that hyperaggregability of platelets was unrelated to the severity of migraine. Deshmukh and Meyer (1976) reported that aggregation increased during the prodromal phase of migraine and diminished during headache. They considered that this could account for the elevation and depression of plasma serotonin in the two phases of migraine but it would seem more likely that the relationship is the other way round since serotonin levels have been estimated in relation to platelet counts. Platelet aggregation may well play a part in the transient neurological deficit of migraine. Permanent deficit appears to be caused by an additional factor of hypercoagulability of the blood (Kalendovsky and Austin, 1975).

Acetylcholine

Acetylcholine causes vasodilation by relaxing arterioles, and the conjunctival vessels become particularly sensitive to its action during migraine headache (Ostfeld et al., 1957). Kunkle (1959) found that acetylcholine was present in CSF samples of 4 out of 14 patients with cluster headache, in one patient with atypical migraine, but not in 7 patients with typical migraine. Migraine cannot be induced by injection of acetylcholine or metacholine (Ostfeld, 1960). There is thus no evidence at the moment to implicate acetylcholine in migraine.

Histamine

Blood histamine levels increase during migraine headache, the mean values in μg/ml being 0·039 before headache, 0·042 during headache and 0·048 24 hours after headache (Anthony and Lance, 1971). The corresponding values in μmol/l are 0·35, 0·38 and 0·43. The post-headache level is significantly higher than the pre-headache level. This correlates with the observation of Sicuteri (1963) that mast cells are degranulated on the side of migraine headache. The injection of histamine into the carotid artery provokes pain but considerably less so than bradykinin. The histamine-liberating substance 48/80 causes intense pain when injected into the external carotid artery (Sicuteri, 1967). Histamine may therefore contribute to the local inflammatory response and vasodilatation of migraine. As described in Chapter 1, the action of histamine depends mainly on histamine-2 receptors in the external carotid circulation (Glover, Carroll and Latt, 1973) but requires both types of receptor for its action on the intracranial vessels.

Bradykinin

Bradykinin is a nonapeptide which has a vasodilator and hypotensive action. It is released from an inactive alpha 2-globulin precursor, kininogen, by proteolytic enzymes in the blood, the plasma kallikreins. Plasma kininogen is diminished at the end of the migraine attack (Sicuteri, Fanciullacci and Anselmi, 1963; Sjaastad, 1970) and a bradykinin-releasing enzyme is increased at the time of headache (Sicuteri, Fanciullacci and Anselmi, 1963). Kinins increase in venous blood during episodes of migraine (Sjaastad, 1970). The injection of bradykinin, 250—500 ng, into the internal carotid artery of man causes pain in the jaw, face, orbital and temporal areas on the side injected (by direct chemical stimulation, not secondary to vasodilatation). Injection of serotonin, 50—100 μg, into a hand vein potentiates greatly the pain-producing effect of bradykinin injected into the same vein.

The intradermal injection of bradykinin into the temporal area causes transient local pain but does not reproduce vascular headache (Elkind, Friedman and Grossman, 1964). The intravenous infusion of bradykinin in man does not cause headache (Fox *et al.*, 1961). The flushing attacks of some cases of carcinoid tumour and the dumping syndrome are caused by increase in circulating bradykinin, but are not associated with headache. Systemic effects of bradykinin are therefore less likely to be of importance in migraine than reactions to its local release. Chapman *et al.* (1960) found a bradykinin-like substance present in the tissues around dilated extracranial vessels during migraine and called it 'neurokinin'. The pain-sensitivity of migrainous vessels could thus be explained by the combined effects of serotonin adsorbed to the vessel wall, the release of histamine from mast cells and the local formation of bradykinin.

Catecholamines

Hsu *et al.* (1976) studied patients whose headaches awakened them from sleep, commonly from the REM phase of sleep. Plasma noradrenaline was significantly elevated in the three hours preceding awakening in those with migraine compared with the same three hours in those who did not awaken with migraine. Once the headache is established, plasma levels of noradrenaline decline and reach a minimum 1½ hours before the peak of migraine headache and then rise as the headache intensity eases (Fog-Møller, Genefke and Bryndum, 1976).

Noradrenaline constricts arterioles and capillaries in the conjunctiva. The sensitivity of these vessels to the topical application of noradrenaline increases in the phase of visual disturbance preceding migraine and diminishes during headache (Ostfeld and Wolff, 1955). Wolff gave intravenous infusions of noradrenaline to migrainous patients at a rate sufficient to cause constriction of the conjunctival vessels and reduce pulsation of the extracranial arteries. When the infusion took place at the height of headache, the headache usually diminished and gradually disappeared. When noradrenaline was infused in headache-free periods for up to 3 hours and then stopped, no headache ensued, showing that migraine headache is not simply a rebound phenomenon following tissue ischaemia (Wolff, 1972).

The part played by catecholamines in the mechanism of migraine must remain open to question at the moment.

Mono-amine oxidase (MAO)

Sicuteri *et al.* (1972) have sought to relate the periodic fluctuation in susceptibility to migraine to the MAO activity of blood platelets which is lower than that of control subjects and reaches its lowest level on the last day of migraine headache or the following day. Sandler *et al*. (1970) have also reported that MAO activity was diminished in 4 patients during an attack of migraine. Recently Sandler, Youdim and Hanington (1974) showed a defect of both phenylethylamine and tyramine metabolism by mono-amine oxidase (types A and B, respectively). This apparent deficit is harder to understand when in our own experience, MAO inhibitors benefit patients with migraine.

AN ATTEMPTED SYNTHESIS

Whatever metabolic changes are implicated in the pathogenesis of migraine, the result is expressed as headache and changes in extra and intracranial blood-flow, as well as more subtle alterations in neuronal activity. The cranial vascular system may thus be regarded as the most conspicuous end organ of the migrainous process. Blood is shunted away from the periphery, giving rise to pallor in the case of the extracranial vascular tree and focal neurological symptoms from cortical ischaemia in the case of the intracranial vessels (*Figure 11.1*). Russell (1973) suggested that this might be a mechanism by which the brain protects itself from harmful metabolites or other harmful chemical agents. In those patients who experience a slow march of fortification spectra or paraesthesiae, the additional factor of the spreading depression of Leão may be evoked by impaired blood supply to the cortex (Milner, 1958).

Extracranial arteries from non-migrainous subjects contract and dilate when they are studied *in vitro* after being removed at operation. It may take hours for spontaneous contraction of strips of the superficial temporal artery to settle down sufficiently to enable the effects of vasoactive amines to be studied on a relatively stable baseline. It is probable that there is a familial tendency toward enhanced vascular contractility in migrainous patients although this has never been demonstrated directly. In that event, jarring of the vessels caused by a direct blow to the head may be sufficient to initiate the sequence of constriction and dilatation which is an integral part of the migraine attack.

Physical exertion or the ingestion of food or drugs which dilate both large and small vessels in a normal subject give rise to a healthy flush and a hyperactive circulation. In a migrainous patient, they may bring about an inappropriate and inco-ordinate circulatory response with constriction of small vessels and dilatation of arteries and veins. Some trigger factors such as stress may operate through a more complex mechanism involving the autonomic nervous system and the release of

humoral agents such as serotonin from body stores. Serotonin is a
potent constrictor of the extracranial circulation in man (Carroll,
Ebeling and Glover, 1974; Lance, Anthony and Gonski, 1967). It has
been postulated that serotonin released from platelets in migraine causes
vasoconstriction and may then be adsorbed to the vessel wall, combining.
with the effects of histamine and kinins to increase pain sensitivity of
the affected arteries. The drop in plasma level after adsorption and

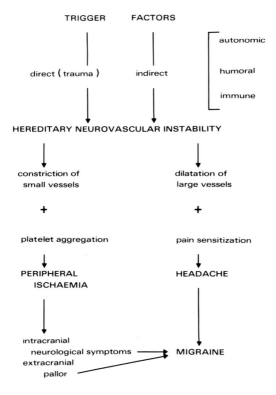

Figure 11.1 Factors in the pathogenesis of migraine

metabolism of released serotonin diminishes a tonic constrictor effect
which would normally tend to counteract any dilator substances such
as histamine, bradykinin and PGE_1. Increased platelet aggregation
reported during migraine may enhance the peripheral ischaemia resulting
from vasoconstriction. The accumulation of lactic acid during the phase
of cerebral ischaemia could also cause a reactive hyperaemia, unopposed

by the normal humoral vasoconstrictive mechanism. The factor responsible for releasing serotonin is unknown but free fatty acids which have this potential are known to be increased in plasma during migraine. The possibility of immune complexes must also be considered since IgG (but not IgA, IgE or IgM) can aggregate and release serotonin from human platelets (Henson and Spiegelberg, 1973). Lord and Duckworth (1977) have shown that mean IgG, IgA and IgM levels are increased in migrainous patients when compared with controls, and demonstrated changes in complement suggesting activation of the classic pathway for delayed hypersensitivity. Immune complexes are deposited in the blood vessels of rabbits when agents which increase vascular permeability or which liberate vasoactive amines from their storage sites are infused (Dalessio, 1976). The cranial arteries of man may thus be a target for immune responses which initiate the migrainous process.

Irrespective of the role of metabolic, humoral or immunological changes in the genesis of migraine, some explanation must be found for the asymmetry of the process, since headache and focal neurological symptoms usually implicate one side more than the other. It has often been suggested that malalignment of the cervical vertebrae or osteophytes growing from them may damage or irritate the nerve plexus surrounding the vertebral artery, giving rise to 'migraine cervicale'. If this were the case, one would expect migraine to be more common in men who are more subject to trauma of the head and neck, and to increase in incidence as age progresses. In fact migraine is more common in women, with its greater prevalence during the reproductive years of life. The involvement of an extracranial artery in a laceration of the scalp may lead to post-traumatic migraine with painful dilatation of the damaged artery. This brings up the possibility of the carotid and vertebral arteries or their branches being compressed at some point in their course, perhaps by over-contraction of muscles in tense persons or an abnormal posture of the head and neck during sleep, to render that part of the vascular tree more reactive to changes in humoral agents, a form of denervation hypersensitivity. I have looked for angiographic evidence that migraine is such an 'entrapment vasculopathy' but so far have found none. The reason for selective involvement of parts of the vascular tree in migraine remains obscure.

The demonstration of metabolic changes of cerebral ischaemia in migraine has led to the hypothesis that the increased cerebral perfusion of the headache phase may simply be a reactive hyperaemia. This explanation is unsatisfying since cases of 'migraine equivalent' may have symptoms of severe and prolonged cortical ischaemia without any headache ensuing and many cases of classic migraine may have a relatively mild headache component. On the other hand, common or non-classic migraine may consist of an intensely severe headache without any focal neurological symptoms. The foregoing argument presupposes that headache is proportional to increase in cerebral blood-flow, which is by no means certain. Cerebral blood-flow greater than that recorded in migraine headache may occur after carbon dioxide inhalation or papaverine injection without causing headache. Moreover Hachinski *et al.* (1976) have reported that 2 out of 4 migrainous patients did not have a significant change in cerebral blood-flow during migraine headache. Abnormal CT scans suggestive of ischaemic cerebral changes, unsuspected cortical infarction and cerebral atrophy have recently been reported in migrainous patients, supporting the concept of peripheral vasoconstriction being responsible for focal neurological symptoms and signs, but the problem of the headache itself has not been resolved. Present evidence supports the view of Wolff and his colleagues that the extracranial circulation is more important as a source of pain in migraine than the intracranial circulation.

Sicuteri (1976) considers that the vascular theory of headache ignores more than it explains. He proposes that cerebral serotonin deficiency lowers the pain threshold and that headache may be of central origin, determined genetically by a derangement of metabolism of brainstem mono-amines, serotonin in particular. The dilatation of vessels then becomes a complementary but inessential component, Fanciullacci, Franchi and Sicuteri (1974) studied the effect of lysergic acid diethylamide (LSD-25) and psilocybin in 2 groups of 36 patients with migraine and other 'essential headaches' compared with 30 normal subjects who did not suffer from headache. Perceptual distortions or hallucinations were experienced by 18 per cent of each headache group and by none of the normal controls with the dosage employed. This suggests that the blood-brain barrier is diminished in headache patients or that they possess unusually sensitive central receptors for these drugs. It is refreshing to have our attention directed once again to the central nervous system and the undoubted changes in neuronal transmission which take place in migraine and related forms of headache but it is difficult to believe that a unilateral headache with its localized vascular concomitants can be entirely determined centrally. A heightened central sensitivity to afferent stimuli, including light, sound and often smells, is an important aspect of the migrainous process but heightened sensitivity to pain of the peripheral apparatus, the vascular end-organ, must surely be essential for the perception of vascular distension as headache.

Migraine appears to be associated with a number of metabolic defects, each of which is a potential danger to the central nervous system. It appears that the late Harold G. Wolff at the time of his death was developing the hypothesis that migraine is an exaggerated adaptive response (Goodell, 1975). Migraine can be regarded as a heightened neurovascular reaction to any rapid change in the internal or external environment, possibly a distorted protective response to any real or imagined threat to the integrity of the brain

CONCLUSIONS

The migraine spectrum includes classic migraine with neurological prodromes, an intermediate form in which neurological symptoms occur during the headache phase, and common migraine. Established facts about migraine may be considered under the following headings: the individual (family history and personality), trigger factors, neurological and vascular phenomena, metabolic changes and the source of pain.

Psychological tests show that migrainous patients are more anxious, sensitive, more easily frustrated and react more to stress than control subjects. They are also more susceptible to hallucinogenic drugs. Undeniable trigger factors for some patients are emotional stress, relaxation after nervous tension, physical exertion, head injury, hormonal fluctuations, hypoglycaemia and some alcoholic drinks. The specificity of certain foods, changes in barometric pressure and other factors has yet to be determined. In many patients there are no obvious precipitating factors.

Unexplained neurological symptoms preceding migraine headache in some patients by as much as 24 hours include mood changes, drowsiness, hunger and thirst, suggesting a hypothalamic disturbance. Other neurological symptoms preceding or accompanying migraine headache may well be secondary to changes in the vertebrobasilar and carotid circulations.

Documented vascular changes comprise phases of diminished cerebral blood-flow, focal or generalized, followed by increased blood-flow, the increased flow not necessarily being accompanied by headache. The most likely explanation is the shunting of blood away from the periphery, the skin in the case of the external carotid circulation, the cortex and brainstem in the case of internal carotid and vertebrobasilar circulations. Cortical ischaemia may result from the constriction of small vessels, platelet aggregation or both. The increased blood-flow which follows may be a reactive hyperaemia or may depend upon specific vasodilator agents.

Metabolic changes in migraine include sodium and fluid retention, abnormal handling of glucose, elevation of free fatty acids, release of serotonin from platelets, elevation of blood noradrenaline before the headache, elevation of blood histamine after the attack, and increased blood ammonia levels in some cases of migraine stupor. Many documented changes involve vasoactive substances which may play a part in altering cerebral blood-flow.

The pain of migraine headache has been attributed to vascular distension and increased sensitivity of the vessel wall. This still seems to be the most important factor in spite of ingenious hypotheses implicating increased central sensitivity to pain impulses.

Migraine may be considered as a hypersensitive protective mechanism for preserving the integrity of the brain against any sudden change in the internal or external environment. The intrinsic reactivity of cranial blood vessels may be sufficiently sensitive to jarring to cause migraine as a direct response to trauma. More commonly, external trigger factors, physical or emotional, operate through the autonomic nervous system, humoral agents or immune mechanisms. Intrinsic bodily rhythms such as the oscillating levels of female hormones may alter vascular sensitivity directly or through humoral mediators. The end result is a neurovascular reaction which reduces the blood supply to vulnerable parts of the brain with results detrimental to the patient. The headache itself, like any form of pain which signals a threat to bodily function, may be a by-product of such reactions even though it represents the major problem to the patient.

REFERENCES

Adams, C.W.M., Orton, C.C. and Zilkha, K.J. (1968). Arterial catecholamine and enzyme histochemistry in migraine. *J. Neurol. Neurosurg. Psychiat.* **31**, 50

Adams, F. (1844). *The Seven Books of Paulus Aegineta*, p. 350. London: Sydenham Society

Anthony, M. (1976). Plasma free fatty acids and prostaglandin E_1 in migraine and stress. *Headache* **16**, 58

Anthony, M. (1977). The role of free fatty acids in migraine. Paper delivered at First International Migraine Symposium, London

Anthony, M., Hinterberger, H. and Lance, J.W. (1967). Plasma serotonin in migraine and stress. *Archs Neurol.* **16**, 544

Anthony, M., Hinterberger, H. and Lance, J.W. (1968). The possible relationship of serotonin to the migraine syndrome. *Res. clin. Stud. Headache* **2**, 29

Anthony, M. and Lance, J.W. (1971). Histamine and serotonin in cluster headache. *Archs. Neurol.* **25**, 225

Anthony, M. and Lance, J.W. (1975). The role of serotonin. In *Modern Topics in Migraine.* Ed J. Pearce, p. 107. London: Heinemann

Appenzeller, O., Davison, K. and Marshall, J. (1963). Reflex vasomotor abnormalities in the hands of migrainous subjects. *J. Neurol. Neurosurg. Psychiat.* **26**, 447

Barrie, M. and Jowett, A. (1967). A pharmacological investigation of cerebro-spinal fluid from patients with migraine. *Brain* **90**, 785

Blau, J.N. and Davis, E. (1970). Small blood-vessels in migraine. *Lancet* **2**, 740

Cahen, R.L. (1974). Emetic effect of biogenic amines. *Res. clin. Stud. Headache* **3**, 227

Carlson, L.A., Ekelund, L-G and Orö, L. (1968). Clinical and metabolic effects of different doses of prostaglandin E_1 in man. *Acta med. scand.* **183**, 423

Carroll, P.R., Ebeling, P.W. and Glover, W.E. (1974). The responses of the human temporal and rabbit ear artery to 5-hydroxytryptamine and some of its antagonists. *Aust. J. exp. Biol. med Sci.* **52**, 813

Chapman, L.F., Ramos, A.O., Goodell, H., Silverman, G. and Wolff, H.G. (1960) A humoral agent implicated in vascular headache of the migrainous type. *Archs. Neurol.* **3**, 223

Couch, J.R. and Hassenein, R.S. (1976). Platelet aggregability in migraine and relation of aggregability to clinical aspects of migraine. *Neurology* **26**, 348

Cumings, J.N. (1971). In *Background to Migraine*, Fourth British Migraine Symposium. p. 76. London: Heinemann

Curran, D.A., Hinterberger, H. and Lance, J.W. (1965). Total plasma serotonin, 5-hydroxyindoleacetic acid and p-hydroxy-m-methoxymandelic acid excretion in normal and migrainous subjects. *Brain* **88**, 997

Curzon, G., Barrie, M. and Wilkinson, M.I.P. (1969). Relationship between headache and amine changes after administration of reserpine to migrainous patients. *J. Neurol. Neurosurg. Psychiat.* **32**, 555

Dalessio, D.J. (1976). The relationship of vasoactive substances to vascular perm-eability, and their role in migraine. *Res. clin. Stud. Headache* **4**, 76

Deshmukh, S.V. and Meyer, J.S. (1976). Cyclic changes in platelet dynamics in migraine. *Neurology* **26**, 347

De Silva, K.L., Ron, M.A. and Pearce, J. (1974). Blood sugar response to glucagon in migraine. *J. Neurol. Neurosurg. Psychiat.* **37**, 105

Downey, J.A., and Frewin, D.B. (1972). Vascular responses in the hands of patients suffering from migraine. *J. Neurol. Neurosurg. Psychiat.* **35**, 258

Dvilansky, A., Rishpon, S., Nathan, I., Zolotow, Z. and Korczyn, A.D. (1976). Release of platelet 5-hydroxytryptamine by plasma taken from patients during and between migraine attacks. *Pain* **2**, 315

Elkind, A.H., Friedman, A.P. and Grossman, J. (1964). Cutaneous blood flow in vascular headache of the migrainous type. *Neurology, Minneap.* **14**, 24

Fanciullacci, M., Franchi, G. and Sicuteri, F. (1974). Hypersensitivity to lysergic acid diethylamide (LSD-25) and psilocybin in essential headache. *Experientia* **30**, 1441

Fog-Møller, F., Genefke, I.K. and Bryndum, B. (1976). Changes in concentration of catecholamines in blood during spontaneous migraine attacks and reserpine induced attacks. *Abstracts International Symposium* Sept. 16–17, p. 10, London: Migraine Trust

Fox, R.H., Goldsmith, R., Kidd, D.J. and Lewis, G.P. (1961). Bradykinin as a vasodilator in man. *J. Physiol. Lond.* **157**, 589

French, E.B., Lassers, B.W. and Desai, M.G. (1967). Reflex vasomotor responses in the hands of migrainous subjects. *J. Neurol. Neurosurg. Psychiat.* **30**, 276

Glover, W.E., Carroll, P.R. and Latt, N. (1973). Histamine receptors in human temporal and rabbit ear arteries. In *International Symposium on Histamine H_2 Receptor Antagonists.* p. 169. Welwyn Garden City: Smith, Kline and French

Goltman, A.M. (1935/36). The mechanism of migraine. *J. Allergy* **7**, 351

Goodell, H. (1975). Evolution of the concept of neurokinin in migraine headache. In *Vasoactive Substances Relevant to Migraine.* Ed. S. Diamond, D.J. Dalessio, T.R. Graham and J.L. Medina. p. 30. Springfield: Thomas

Graham, J.R. and Wolff, H.G. (1938). Mechanism of migraine headache and action of ergotamine tartrate. *Archs Neurol. Psychiat., Chicago* **39**, 737

Grant, E.C.G. (1965). Relation of arterioles in the endometrium to headache from oral contraceptives. *Lancet* **1**, 1143

Hachinski, V.C., Norris, J.W., Cooper, P.W. and Edmeads, J.G. (1976). Cerebral hemodynamics in the migraine syndrome. *Neurology* **4**, 390

Hauptmann, A. (1946). Capillaries in the finger nail fold in patients with neurosis, epilepsy and migraine. *Archs Neurol. Psychiat., Chicago* **56**, 631

Henson, P.M. and Spiegelberg (1973). Release of serotonin from human platelets induced by aggregated immunoglobulins of different classes and sub-classes. *J. Clin. Invest.* **52**, 1282

Heyck, H. (1969). Pathogenesis of migraine. In *Res. clin. Stud. Headache.* Vol 2, p. 1

Hilton, B.P. and Cumings, J.N. (1971). An assessment of platelet aggregation induced by 5-hydroxytryptamine. *J. clin. Path.,* **24**, 250

Hilton, B.P. and Cumings, J.N. (1972). 5-hydroxytryptamine level and platelet aggregation responses in subjects with acute migraine headache. *J. Neurol. Neurosurg. Psychiat.* **35**, 505

Hockaday, J.M., Macmillan, A.L. and Whitty, C.W.M. (1967). Vasomotor-reflex response in idiopathic and hormone-dependent migraine. *Lancet* **1**, 1023

Hockaday, J.M., Williamson, D.H. and Whitty, C.W.M. (1971). Blood glucose levels and fatty acid metabolism in migraine related to fasting. *Lancet* **1**, 1153

Hsu, L.G.U., Crisp, A.H., Koval, J., Kalucy, R.S., Chen, C.N., Carruthers, M. and Zilkha, K. (1976). Electroencephalogram and plasma levels of catecholamines, tryptophan, glucose, insulin, free fatty acids and prostaglandins during sleep preceding early-morning migraine. *International Symposium*, Sept. 16–17, p. 11. London: Migraine Trust

Kalendovsky, Z. and Austin, J.H. (1975). Complicated Migraine: its association with increased platelet aggregability and abnormal plasma coagulation factors. *Headache* **15**, 18

Kimball, R.W. Friedman, A.P. and Vallejo, E. (1960). Effect of serotonin in migraine patients. *Neurology, Minneap.* **10**, 107

Kimball, R.W. and Goodman, M.A. (1966). Effects of reserpine on amino-acid excretion in patients with migraine. *J. Neurol. Neurosurg. Psychiat.* **29**, 190

Kunkle, E.C. (1959). Acetylcholine in the mechanism of headaches of the migraine type. *Archs Neurol. Psychiat., Chicago* **84**, 135

Lance, J.W., Anthony, M. and Gonski, A. (1967). Serotonin, the carotid body and cranial vessels in migraine. *Archs Neurol.* **16**, 553

Lashley, K.S. (1941). Patterns of cerebral integration indicated by the scotomas of migraine. *Archs Neurol. Fsychiat., Chicago* **46**, 331

Lord, G.D.A. and Duckworth, J.W. (1977). Immunoglobulin and complement studies in migraine. *Headache* **17**, 163

Lund, F. (1957). Studies on the shape of the temporal artery pulsations in vascular headache, particularly migraine. *Acta med. scand.* **158**, 21

Macmillan, A.L. and Hockaday, J. (1966). The effect of migraine and ergot upon reflex vasodilatation to radiant heating. *Proc. 4th Europ. Conf. Microcirculation* p. 343. Basel/New York: Karger

Marshall, W.H. (1959). Spreading cortical depression of Leão. *Physiol. Rev.* **39**, 239

McCalden, T.A., Bloom, D. and Rosendorff, C. (1975). The effects of jaundiced plasma and hypercholesterolaemic plasma on vascular sensitivity to injected noradrenaline. *Experientia* **31**, 1173

Milner, P.M. (1958). Note on a possible correspondence between the scotomas of migraine and spreading depression of Leão. *Electroenceph. clin. Neurophysiol.* **10**, 705

Norris, J.W., Hachinski, V.C. and Cooper, P.W. (1975). Changes in cerebral blood-flow during a migraine attack. *Br. med. J.* **3**, 676

Ostfeld, A.M. (1960). Migraine headache: its physiology and biochemistry. *J. Am. Ass.* **174**, 110

Ostfeld, A.M., Chapman, L.F., Goodell, H. and Wolff, H.G. (1957). Summary of evidence concerning a noxious agent active locally during migraine headache. *Psychosom. Med.* **19**, 199

Ostfeld, A.M. and Wolff, H.G. (1955). Studies on headache: Arterenol (norepinephrine) and vascular headache of the migraine type. *Archs. Neurol. Psychiat., Chicago* **74**, 131

Penfield, W. (1932). Operative treatment of migraine and observations on the mechanisms of vascular pain. *Trans. Am. Acad. Ophthal. Oto-lar.* **37**, 50

Rao, N.S. and Pearce, J. (1971). Hypothalamo-pituitary-adrenal axis studies in migraine with special reference to insulin sensitivity. *Brain* **94**, 289

Redisch, W. and Pelzer, R.H. (1943). Capillary studies in migraine: effect of ergotamine tartrate and water diuresis. *Am. Heart. J.* **26**, 598

Russell, A. (1973). The implications of hyperammonaemia in rare and common disorders, including migraine. *Mount Sinai J. Med.* **40**, 723

Sandler, M. (1972). Migraine: a pulmonary disease? *Lancet* **1**, 618

Sandler, M., Youdim, M.B.H., and Hanington, E. (1974). A phenylethylamine oxidasing defect in migraine. *Nature, Lond.* **250**, 335

Sandler, M., Youdim, M.B.H., Southgate, J. and Hanington, E. (1970). The role of tyramine in migraine: some possible biochemical mechanisms. In *Background to Migraine*, Third British Migraine Symposium. p. 103. London: Heinemann

Sicuteri, F. (1963). Mast cells and their active substances. Their role in the pathogenesis of migraine. *Headache* **3**, 86

Sicuteri, F. (1967). Vasoneuroactive substances and their implication in vascular pain. *Res. clin. Stud. Headache* **1**, 6

Sicuteri, F. (1976). Migraine, a central biochemical dysnociception. *Headache* **16**, 145

Sicuteri, F., Buffoni, F., Anselmi, B. and Del Bianco, P.L. (1972). An enzyme (MAO) defect on the platelets in migraine. *Res. clin. Stud. Headache,* **3**, 245

Sicuteri, F., Fanciullacci, M. and Anselmi, B. (1963). Bradykinin release and inactivation in man. *Int. Archs Allergy appl Immun.* **22**, 77

Sicuteri, F., Testi, A. and Anselmi, B. (1961). Biochemical investigations in headache: increase in hydroxyindoleacetic acid excretion during migraine attacks. *Int. Archs Allergy appl. Immun.* **19**, 55

Simard, D. and Paulson, O.B. (1973). Cerebral vasomotor paralysis during migraine attack. *Archs Neurol.* **29**, 206

Sjaastad, O. (1970). Kinin- and histamine-investigations in vascular headache. In *Kliniske Aspekter i Migraeneforskningen* p. 61. Copenhagen: Nordlundes Bogtrykkeri

Skinhøj, E. (1970). Determination of regional cerebral blood-flow within the internal carotid system during the migraine attack. In *Kliniske Aspekter i Migraeneforskningen* p. 43. Copenhagen: Nordlundes Bogtrykkeri

Skinhøj, E. (1973). Hemodynamic studies within the brain during migraine. *Archs Neurol.* **29**, 95

Somerville, B.W. (1976). Platelet-bound and free seretonin levels in jugular and forearm venous blood during migraine. *Neurology* **26**, 41

Southren, A.L., and Christoff, N. (1962). Cerebrospinal fluid serotonin in brain tumour and other neurological disorders determined by a spectrophoto-fluorometric technique. *J. Lab. clin. Med.* **59**, 320

Thonnard-Neumann, E. (1969). Some interrelationships of vasoactive substances and basophilic leukocytes in migraine headache. *Headache* **9**, 130

Thonnard-Neumann, E. and Taylor, W.L. (1968). The basophilic leukocyte and migraine. *Headache* **8**, 98

Tunis, M.M. and Wolff, H.G. (1952). Analysis of cranial artery pulse waves in patients with vascular headache of the migraine type. *Am. J. med. Sci.* **224**, 565

Tunis, M.M. and Wolff, H.G. (1953). Studies on headache: long-term observations of the reactivity of the cranial arteries in subjects with vascular headache of the migraine type. *Archs Neurol. Psychiat., Chicago* **70**, 551

Welch, K.M.A., Chabi, E., Bartosh, L., Achar, U.S., and Meyer, J.S. (1975). Cerebrospinal fluid gamma aminobutyric acid levels in migraine. *Br. med. J.* **3**, 516

Welch, K.M.A., Nell, J. Chabi, E., Mathew, N.T., Neblett, C.R. and Meyer, J.S. (1976). Cyclic nucleotide studies in migraine. *Neurology* **26**, 380

Wennerholm, M. (1961). Postural vascular reactions in cases of migraine and related vascular headaches. *Acta med. scand.* **169**, 131

White, J.C. and Smithwick, R.H. (1944). *The Autonomic Nervous System* p. 255. London: Kimpton

White, J. and Sweet, W. (1955). *Pain. Its Mechanism and Neurosurgical Control.* Springfield: Thomas

Wolff, H.G. (1972). *Headache and Other Head Pain.* Third Edn. Revised by D.J. Dalessio. New York: Oxford University Press

Twelve

The Treatment of Migraine

Willis in 1684 wrote of migraine in a noble lady and stated that 'this Distemper . . . having pitched its tents near the confines of the Brain, had so long besieged its regal tower, yet it had not taken it . . . . There was no kind of Medicines both Cephalicks, Antiscorbuticks, Hysterical, all famous Specificks, which she took not, both from the Learned and the unlearned, from Quacks, and old Women, and yet notwithstanding she professed, that she had received from no Remedy, or method of Curing, any thing of Cure or Ease, but that the Contumacious and rebellious Disease, refused to be tamed, being deaf to the charms of every Medicine.

Much is known about migraine and much can be done for the patient who is subject to it, but there is no complete and satisfying 'cure'. Migraine does not destroy life but can destroy the joy, value and rewards of living. It is a disease which warrants full attention from the general practitioner, who should be the person most qualified to treat it.

If migraine is a distorted protective response to any real or imagined threat to the integrity of the brain as postulated in Chapter 11, it may never be possible to eliminate it completely in all patients. In our present state of knowledge, the management of migraine comprises removing trigger factors whenever possible, stabilizing neurovascular reactions by psychological and physiological means, blocking any humoral mediators known to be involved in migraine, 'splinting' the vascular end-organ pharmacologically to prevent painful vasodilatation, and relieving pain when all else fails.

The treatment of migraine starts while the history is being taken and continues during the physical examination. This gives time for some degree of mutual understanding to be established between doctor and patient, even if the two have never met before. The nature of any precipitating factors and the patient's reaction to them will have been discussed and some assessment made of the patient's psychological state and capacity for physical relaxation. If the history is typical of migraine headache, the patient should be assured that there is no possibility of cerebral tumour or other progressive disease causing his or her symptoms and hence no need for extensive and expensive investigations. If doubt does exist, then reassurance and management will have to await the outcome of a logical sequence of investigations as described in Chapter 15.

Once a careful history is taken, it may be possible to identify certain trigger factors which can be eliminated. Intelligent patients will already be avoiding situations which they have found readily provoke an attack. They will have ceased sleeping in on Sunday mornings, taking strenuous exercise on a hot day, missing meals, drinking red wine or eating certain foods which they are convinced do not agree with them.

Psychological management

There is an important role in psychological counselling for the doctor of first contact who ideally knows the patient in his or her family setting and is in the best position to give advice. Sometimes patients will discuss embarrassing personal problems more freely with an outsider, a consultant physician, neurologist or psychiatrist, than they would with a doctor who knows them and their family socially. Such a discussion takes time and tolerance and may not necessarily find solutions for the problems which emerge. In any event, it gives patients a chance to unburden themselves, the opportunity to gain objective advice, and the knowledge that their problem is not unique and has been overcome by many others. Manipulation of the patient's personality or life pattern is not always possible but the very fact of free discussion helps the patient and gives confidence that the doctor understands that he is dealing with an individual. It may be possible for patients to arrange their daily routine by reducing peak periods of stress and redistributing their work load. The object is to make any change gradually, to smooth out the peaks and troughs of life as far as possible and to adjust happily to those fluctuations which will inevitably remain. Migrainous patients are not subject to more stress than the general population but they react more forcibly to stress. The external environment can be stabilized to some extent and then patients must concentrate on themselves and their reactions to change. Friedman (1970) said of one of his patients that he 'has an occupation that takes him through the world from the Himalayas in Tibet to Somaliland, indeed from the highest altitudes to the lowest, from the wettest to the driest – experiencing climatic, food and cultural changes. But his migraine remains, for he carries his personal environment with him.'

Building up resistance to stress from within can use both psychological and physiological techniques. Mitchell and Mitchell (1971) compared two such programmes. In the first programme, relaxation training was followed by the application of this training to the tension-producing situation peculiar to that individual. The second treatment group went on to desensitization procedures which included making a graded list of anxiety-provoking stimuli, evoking these by imagery, and pairing each stimulus with a relaxed state. A further stage was 'assertive therapy' in which the subjects underwent training in acting out their feelings of love, affection or hostility in socially acceptable and appropriate forms. Various difficulties such as sexual problems were explained and discussed. While the level of anxiety did not drop appreciably during the 32-week treatment period, the last group with combined relaxation, desensitization and assertive therapy showed significant reduction in the frequency and severity of migraine compared with the other group.

With the object of training patients to increase their stress threshold, Mitchell and White (1976) have introduced a programme of 'behavioural self-management' in which patients identify and analyse problems in their personal environment and behaviour, to work out their own management strategy and to apply self-control techniques.

Physiological management (relaxation and biofeedback)

Simple relaxation training, as described in Chapter 9, can be applied to migrainous patients to reduce the frequency and severity of headache. Warner and Lance (1975) found that four sessions of training in conjunction with an outpatients' clinic caused improvement which persisted for 6 months in 8 of 12 patients.

Relaxation training is often augmented by feedback from an electromyogram (EMG) of the frontal and temporal muscles, from skin temperatures of scalp and hand, or from recordings of the temporal artery pulsations. Spontaneous recovery from migraine headache is associated with an increase in blood-flow and skin temperature in the hands. Sargent, Green and Walters (1972) trained patients to increase skin temperatures in the hands in relation to the forehead and to use this technique to abort headaches. Of 62 migrainous patients who carried out the treatment programme, 74 per cent improved. It is very difficult to find valid controls for a technique which relies on auto-suggestion but various forms of 'autogenic feedback training' are now being studied. Medina, Diamond and Franklin (1976) have combined skin temperature and EMG feedback. Koppman and his colleagues (1974) have shown that it was possible for 7 out of 9 migrainous patients to control the amplitude of pulsation of their temporal arteries after 2 to 4 weeks of training for 2 to 3 hourly sessions each week. It remains to be seen whether this can be applied to the suppression of migraine headache.

Price and Tursky (1976) divided 40 migrainous patients and 40 control subjects into 4 treatment groups. The first group was exposed to feedback of hand temperature, the second group to false feedback, the third to relaxation procedures and the fourth to a 'neutral' tape of instructions on how to grow an avocado plant. The most dramatic change of any group was observed among the avocado-growers who developed vasoconstriction in the hands! The other three treatments produced a small increase in blood-flow in normal controls but no significant change in the migrainous patients. Temporal artery pulsations increased in normal subjects but diminished in migraine sufferers. This study confirms that vascular responses are abnormal in migraine and emphasizes that further studies of conditioning procedures are necessary before skin temperature biofeedback is widely applied to the treatment of migraine.

Transcendental meditation and hypnotherapy

Any means of achieving emotional equilibrium and physical relaxation might be expected to be helpful in migraine. It was therefore disappointing to learn that transcendental meditation was of benefit to only 6 of 17 patients studied by Benson, Klemchuk and Graham (1974).

The results of hypnotherapy are more encouraging. Anderson, Basker and Dalton (1975) compared 23 patients undergoing hypnotherapy with a control group of 24 treated with prochlorperazine. The hypnosis group (in 6 sessions at intervals of 10 to 14 days) were given 'ego-strengthening' suggestions that they would have less tension, anxiety and apprehension as well as specific suggestions about constricting the arteries in their heads. Patients were asked to practise hypnosis daily and to use it to abort a threatened attack of migraine. The trial extended for 12 months in the last 3 months of which 43·5 per cent of the hypnotherapy group were free of headache, compared with

12·5 per cent of controls. The median number of attacks per month dropped from 4·5 to 0·5 in the patients treated with hypnosis compared with 3·3 to 2·9 in the prochlorperazine group.

Acupuncture

Acupuncture has been practised in China for more than 2000 years and is currently enjoying a vogue in the western world. A report by Kajdos (1975) stated that headaches were relieved in 136 of 309 patients after 8 to 10 sessions. Another 128 patients improved and only 45 remained unchanged. My own experience has been that patients improve while undergoing treatment and relapse shortly thereafter.

Exercise

Standing on the head improves vasoconstrictor reflexes in scalp arteries (Wolff, 1963) and has a rational basis for the gymnastically adroit, but is of limited application.

Hormones

Hormonal factors are of importance in migraine and the use of progestogenic agents and injections of chorionic gonadotrophin have been recommended in treatment. In 1962, Lundberg reported that 55 of 84 patients (including 6 men) became free of migraine attacks when treated with methylnortestosterone, 1–2 mg daily, or allyloestrenol, 2·5–15 mg daily, given for 3 weeks of the menstrual cycle, or continuously. Continuous administration caused amenorrhoea in most cases. Menstrual disturbances occurred in 36 out of 76 women with cyclical therapy and 9 noticed hirsuties, acne or hoarseness. We followed up this report by using allyloestrenol in the dosage recommended in a pilot trial of 20 patients. The results were disappointing and did not warrant the organization of a controlled trial. Another progestogenic agent, flumedroxone, the use of which had also been advocated by Lundberg, was subjected to a controlled trial in which its effect was compared with that of methysergide over a period of 9 months in 35 patients (Hudgson, Foster and Newell, 1967). There was no significant difference between the number of attacks per month experienced before the trial period and the number of monthly attacks while taking flumedroxone. This contrasted with the improvement of all but 3 patients taking methysergide.

Gonadotrophic hormone has been used in the treatment of migraine for more than 30 years. We have given gonadotrophic hormone 500 I.U. twice weekly to 26 patients for periods of 2 to 10 months. Only 10 showed worthwhile improvement and it was felt that this result, which may well have been due to the natural history of the disease, did not warrant the trouble and expense of regular injections.

Various forms of contraceptive pill make migraine worse in most instances, and permanent neurological deficit has been reported in patients whose vasoconstrictive phase of migraine was prolonged while taking oral contraceptives.

The only hormonal treatment which is at least 60 per cent effective is pregnancy.

Prevention of salt and water retention

Fluid retention is common for several days before the menstrual period and is also common immediately before migraine headache. The fact that menstruation and migraine often coincide led to the use of salt restriction and diuretics in the treatment of migraine whether or not it tended to occur with the menses. Fluid retention may indeed be prevented by such measures but migraine usually continues unabated.

Histamine desensitization

Histamine, given by incrementing subcutaneous injections or weekly intravenous infusions, has been used in the treatment of migraine for many years. This is a difficult procedure to adapt to a controlled trial to see whether it really is effective. A follow-up for 8 months after a course of 3 intravenous infusions at weekly intervals revealed that 21 per cent of patients became headache-free and another 42 per cent were more than half-improved (Selby and Lance, 1960). It is not known whether this treatment has some non-specific effect on vascular reactivity, or whether its action is purely psychological.

Manipulative and surgical procedures

Success has been claimed for manipulation of the neck in the treatment of migraine headache as in many other fields, but objective evidence is lacking. Cyriax (1962) stated that 'an attack of migraine can sometimes be instantly aborted by strong traction on the neck. Half a minute's traction in some cases is regularly successful, in others not. The mechanism is obscure (it may be connected with the stretching of the carotid and vertebral arteries) and the phenomenon would clearly repay further study . . .'. Cyriax goes on to say 'A minority of patients have reported to me, some years after the reduction by manipulation of a cervical disc, that since that time attacks of obvious migraine have ceased'. Such improvement has only been noted in middle-aged patients, not in the young, and Cyriax postulates that pressure by osteophytes on the vertebral artery and the nerve plexus surrounding it may therefore play some part in the production of migraine. Since many patients have already undergone cervical manipulation without success by the time they are referred to a neurologist, the author remains sceptical, although prepared to alter his views should any controlled observations be published. The author wonders whether manipulating the neck is really a sophisticated way of pulling the patient's leg.

Surgical procedures were discussed in the previous chapter and it was concluded that operations on sympathetic or parasympathetic nerve pathways, and ligation of branches of the external carotid or middle meningeal arteries or both did not provide any lasting benefit. A new surgical approach has been described by Cook (1973) who has applied cryosurgery to scalp arteries on the side affected by headache in 322 migrainous patients. He reported a six-month follow-up of 106 patients of whom 57 stated that they had experienced a reduction of attacks by 75 per cent or more since the procedure.

Pharmacotherapy

The drug treatment of migraine falls into the following categories:
(1) Drugs which constrict the extracranial arteries such as ergotamine tartrate, dihydroergotamine, and 1-methylergotamine hydrogen tartrate (MY25). Serotonin and noradrenaline have also been used experimentally for this purpose.
(2) Serotonin antagonists, some of which simulate the action of serotonin in potentiating the effect of vasoconstrictor agents: methysergide (Deseril, Sansert), cyproheptadine (Periactin), pizotifen (BC105, Sandomigran), methylergol carbamide maleate (Lysenyl).
(3) Drugs blocking beta-adrenergic receptors on blood vessels, thereby diminishing vasodilator responses, e.g. propranolol (Inderal).

(4) Drugs which block central vasomotor reflexes and diminish vascular reactivity such as clonidine (Catapres, Dixarit).

(5) Mono-amine oxidase inhibitors, such as phenelzine (Nardil), which permit the accumulation of serotonin and other vasoactive amines such as noradrenaline.

(6) A miscellaneous group including anticonvulsants, such as carba-mazepine (Tegretol); indomethacin (Indocid, Indocin); and methdilazine (Tacaryl, Dilosyn), which has anti-bradykinin properties.

PHARMACEUTICAL AGENTS EMPLOYED IN THE TREATMENT OF MIGRAINE

The objects of drug therapy in migraine are to assist the psychological and physiological adjustment of the patient, to prevent excessive dilatation of the extracranial arteries without reducing cerebral blood-flow and to block the action of humoral mediators such as serotonin and histamine which are thought to play a part in the migrainous process.

Ergotamine

Ergotamine tartrate has been used as a specific agent for the treatment of acute attacks of migraine for about fifty years. The fast phase of its elimination half-life is 5 to 6 hours (Meier and Schreier, 1976). Saxena (1972) demonstrated that it constricts the external carotid circulation of the dog much more readily than other arteries including the vetebral. We have found a similar selective action in the monkey circulation (Spira, Mylecharane and Lance, 1976). The injection of 3.6 $\mu g/kg$ intravenously (equivalent to 0.25 mg in a 70-kg man) increased resistance in the external carotid artery by 90 per cent compared with a non-specific increase of 27 per cent in the internal carotid artery. External carotid arterial constriction reached its peak 2 to 11 minutes after administration and was well maintained during a 2-hour period of observation. There was no significant change in systemic blood pressure.

Aellig and Berde (1969) have shown that the vasoconstrictor activity of ergotamine compounds depends upon the pre-existing vascular resistance. Working with the perfused dog hind-limb they found that ergotamine, dihydroergotamine (DHE) and 1-methylergotamine (MY25) act as vasoconstrictors when the vascular resistance is low but are transformed into vasodilators as the vascular resistance is increased.

Berde (1972) emphasized the possible significance of capacitance vessels in the microcirculation, the part of the venous compartment which follows the postcapillary resistance vessels. Low frequency sympathetic nerve stimulation increases the tone of the capacitance vessels and higher frequencies also contract the resistance vessels, particularly the precapillary resistance vessels. Ergotamine and dihydro-ergotamine have no effect on the precapillary sphincters but constrict the capacitance vessels, which decrease the blood content of the area and increase venous return. Hydergine (dihydroergocristine, dihydro-ergocornine and dihydroergocryptine) also dilates the precapillary sphincters. The part played by the capacitance vessels in migraine is as yet unknown but there is some evidence that they may be overdistended because of the facial and scalp oedema which has been reported on occasions, and that flow in this system may be slowed down because of blood being shunted away from the periphery. Ergotamine has an antiserotonin action in preventing serotonin-induced oedema of the rat's paw which is much less than that of methysergide but is longer lasting.

Human studies have shown that ergotamine has little or no constrictor action on the cerebral or retinal arteries. The intramuscular injection of doses of 0·25 to 1·0 mg does not alter regional cerebral blood-flow in man (Edmeads, Hachinski and Norris, 1976). Edmeads, Hachinski and Norris conclude their summary of the effects of ergotamine: 'there now appears to be no valid reason to deny even patients with severe vasoconstrictive auras the benefits of ergotamine.'

Methysergide (Deseril, Sansert)

Methysergide (1-methyl-D-lysergic acid butanolamide) is an ergot derivative with a fast elimination half-life of about 3 hours (Meier and Schreier, 1976). It has a serotonin-blocking action but also simulates the effect of serotonin in that it potentiates the vasoconstrictive effect of noradrenaline. It exerts only a mild and transient direct constrictor response on its own. In the monkey circulation, methysergide antagonizes the constrictor effect of serotonin more effectively in the internal than the external carotid circulation by both competitive and non-competitive mechanisms. There is no effect on the dilator responses to histamine, bradykinin or prostaglandin E_1. Small doses of methysergide have been shown to potentiate the external carotid vasoconstrictor effects of noradrenaline in the dog (Saxena, 1972) and monkey (Mylecharane et al., 1977) and in the isolated human temporal artery (Carroll, Ebeling and Glover, 1974).

The application of methysergide solution to the conjunctiva, or the oral administration of methysergide, does not directly constrict the conjunctival vessels but increases their sensitivity to the constrictor effects of noradrenaline (Dalessio *et al.*, 1961).

It is uncertain whether methysergide benefits migraine by reducing the pain-producing action of serotonin which has been released from platelets and has been adsorbed to the vessel wall, or by reducing the vasoconstrictor effects of released serotonin on small arteries, or by maintaining tonic constriction of large arteries once the serotonin level has fallen, or by a combination of these effects.

Methysergide has proven the most useful prophylactic agent in migraine (Curran, Hinterberger and Lance, 1967). Regular medication with methysergide, 2–6 mg daily, suppresses migraine completely in about 26 per cent of patients and improves substantially another 40 per cent (Curran and Lance, 1964). About 40 per cent of patients experience side-effects, chiefly abdominal discomfort and muscle cramps, when treatment is first started but these usually pass off after some days or weeks. Less common side-effects include insomnia, depression, a sensation of swelling in the face or throat, increase in the venules over nose and cheeks and gain in weight (Curran, Hinterberger and Lance, 1967; Curran and Lance, 1964). About 10 per cent of patients are unable to tolerate methysergide because of persistent unpleasant symptoms or the appearance of peripheral vasoconstriction with pallor of the extremities, intermittent claudication, or, very rarely, angina pectoris. These symptoms disappear on ceasing medication or, if mild, may be overcome by combining a vasodilator drug with methysergide (Lance, Fine and Curran, 1963).

Peripheral vascular disease, coronary artery disease, hypertension, a history of thrombophlebitis or peptic ulcer, and pregnancy, are all relative, but not absolute, contra-indications to the use of methysergide. The reason for avoiding methysergide in the first four conditions is fairly clear, since arterial vasoconstriction is a recognized side-effect. The administration of methysergide was found to double basal gastric secretion of hydrochloric acid in patients with peptic ulcer, and hence its use is best avoided in this condition. There is no evidence to suggest that methysergide is harmful to mother or foetus, but it has been our own practice to suspend its use once a patient becomes pregnant because of innate conservatism. Three of our patients continued with methysergide throughout pregnancy and bore normal full-term infants.

Graham (1967) reported that retroperitoneal fibrosis, pleural fibrosis or cardiac valvular fibrosis had developed in about 100 patients of the half-million who were estimated to have been treated with methysergide at that time. In 15 years of using methysergide extensively, I have known 3 patients with retroperitoneal fibrosis, 1 with pleural fibrosis and 1 patient who developed a cardiac murmur while under observation. It must be borne in mind that other agents may cause fibrotic syndromes and that in some cases no cause may be apparent. Lewis *et al*. (1975) reported a retrospective study of 7 patients with retroperitoneal fibrosis from the London Hospital. None had ever taken methysergide but 4 of the 7 had taken excessive amounts of analgesics. Those cases that are associated with methysergide usually resolve completely once treatment is ceased.

The fibrotic complications of methysergide may well be the result of its serotonin-like action. Graham (1967) commented on the similarity of the appearance at operation of valvular fibrosis in methysergide-treated patients to that seen in carcinoid syndrome. The administration of serotonin to rats either decreases or increases granuloma formation, depending upon the function of the adrenal gland (Bianchine and Eade, 1967). Excessive fibrosis appears only if adrenal insufficiency is induced. This raises the question of whether there might be adrenal insufficiency in patients who develop fibrotic syndromes in response to serotonin or methysergide. It is possible that any drug which relies upon a serotonin-simulating action for the treatment of migraine has the potential of producing excessive fibrosis in susceptible subjects.

Pizotifen (Sandomigran), cyproheptadine (Periactin)

Pizotifen is a benzocycloheptathiophene derivative which is structurally similar to cyproheptadine (Periactin) and the tricyclic antidepressants. It has an elimination half-life of about 23 hours (Meier and Schreier, 1976). Pizotifen and cyproheptadine block the constrictor effect of serotonin on the isolated human temporal artery but, unlike methysergide, do not potentiate the effects of noradrenaline. In the monkey circulation pizotifen antagonizes serotonin-induced constriction in the internal carotid artery but, in large doses, actually potentiates the effect of serotonin in the external carotid artery (Mylecharane *et al*., 1977; Spira, Mylecharane and Lance, 1976). Pizotifen blocks the dilator action of histamine in the internal carotid circulation but is considerably less effective in the external carotid system. Extensive clinical trials have demonstrated that pizotifen reduces the frequency and severity of migraine headache in most patients, although it is not as effective as methysergide (Speight and Avery, 1972). The most common side-effects are drowsiness and weight gain from increased appetite. The action and side-effects of cyproheptadine are similar to that of pizotifen although there are few publications concerning its use in migraine (Curran and Lance, 1964; Lance, Anthony and Somerville, 1970).

Cimetidine

Cimetidine is the most recent of a new generation of antihistamines which have been termed histamine-2 blocking agents because they antagonize certain actions of histamine such as the stimulation of gastric acid secretion which are untouched by the antihistamines to which we have become accustomed (now known as histamine-1 blockers). In the monkey, cimetidine blocks the dilator effect of histamine in the external carotid artery but is much less effective in the internal carotid artery (Spira, Mylecharane and Lance, 1976). It does not influence the systemic vasodepressor effect of histamine. By way of contrast, mepyramine (a histamine-1 antagonist), blocks the fall in systemic blood pressure, supplements histamine blockade by cime-tidine in the internal carotid artery but does not appreciably alter its effects on the external carotid circulation. It may be deduced that the external carotid artery of the monkey contains mainly histamine-2 receptors. Similar results have been reported in the dog and in the iso-lated human temporal artery. Cimetidine is now undergoing clinical trial in the management of migraine.

Clonidine (Catapres, Dixarit)

Clonidine, 2- (2,6 - dichlorophenylamino) 2-imidazoline hydrochloride, is a hypotensive agent which is undergoing clinical assessment for the prophylaxis of migraine. Zaimis and Hanington (1969) found that pretreatment with clonidine reduced the vasoconstrictor response of the cat femoral artery to noradrenaline, adrenaline and angiotensin as well as diminishing the vasodilator effect of isoprenaline, so that it appeared to damp down both constrictor and dilator responses by a direct action on the arterial wall not involving alpha- or beta-adrenergic receptors. These results have not been substantiated by our studies in the monkey circulation (Mylecharane et al., 1977), in which clonidine 0·5 and 2 μg/kg potentiated the constrictor effects of serotonin and noradrenaline and the dilator effect of bradykinin. It left unaltered the responses to PGE_1 and histamine. In these doses, which clearly did not reduce the reactivity of the vessels, central effects were observed in that the pressor response to carotid occlusion and the cranial vascular constrictor response to stimulation of the cervical sympathetic trunk were both reduced. Systemic blood pressure rose transiently after the intravenous injection of clonidine, then a long-lasting hypotension ensued.

There have been mixed reports concerning the efficacy of clonidine in migraine. Initial optimistic reports (Barrie *et al.*, 1968; Shafar and Tallett, 1972; Stensrud and Sjaastad, 1976b; Zaimis and Hanington, 1969) have been followed by negative double-blind trials (Ryan and Robert, Jr, 1975; Shaw and Saunders, 1972). Clonidine may find a place in the treatment of sub-groups of migraine, possibly those in whom symptoms of cerebral vasoconstriction are prominent, but this remains to be proved. The tablets are manufactured in doses of 25 and 150 micrograms. The dose advocated for migraine varies from 25 micrograms, twice daily, to 75 micrograms, three times daily.

Beta-adrenergic blocking agents

The dilatation of peripheral arteries in response to adrenaline is mediated by beta-2 receptors in the vessel wall. Beta blockade could therefore prevent vasodilatation in response to any humoral agents employing those receptors. There have been a number of controlled trials which have demonstrated the superiority of propranolol (Inderal) over placebo in the prevention of migraine (Diamond and Medina, 1976; Forssman *et al.*, 1976; Stensrud and Sjaastad, 1976a; Weber and Reinmuth, 1971; Widerøe and Vigander, 1974). Side-effects are mild, occasional postural hypotension and insomnia, but the drug should be avoided in patients with a tendency to bronchospasm. Other beta-blockers, such as practolol and pindolol have not been shown to be of value.

Amitriptyline

Amitriptyline is well known as a tricyclic antidepressant and its use in tension headache has been discussed in Chapter 9. It has been mentioned sporadically as a useful agent in migraine, particularly when there is associated depression. Gomersall and Stuart (1973) confirmed that it was effective in reducing the frequency of migraine headache. In a larger open trial, Couch and his colleagues (1976) found that amitriptyline, most commonly given in doses of 50 to 75 mg daily, produced an

80 per cent improvement in 57 per cent of patients. There was only a weak correlation with pre-existing depression. In our own experience amitriptyline is particularly valuable when frequent migraine attacks are associated with tension headache.

Mono-amine oxidase inhibitors

Since serotonin levels are lowered in migraine, the use of a drug which maintains or increases serotonin levels is a logical form of treatment and a number of favourable reports concerning MAO inhibitors have appeared in the past (Blumenthal and Fuchs, 1963). Anthony and Lance (1969) treated 25 patients, who had failed to respond to other forms of interval medication, with phenelzine, 45 mg daily, for periods up to 2 years. The frequency of headache was reduced to less than half in 20 of the 25 patients. Although mean plasma serotonin increased by about 50 per cent there was no correlation between the serotonin level and response of each individual patient. We have continued to use this form of treatment in patients resistant to other therapy. Patients are issued with a notice stating that they must not have cheese, meat extracts, red wines (or any alcoholic drink in excess), broad beans, pickled herrings, chicken livers (pâté), or any tablets or injections other than those prescribed for their migraine such as aspirin, codeine or ergotamines. They are particularly warned against having injections of pethidine, morphine, reserpine, tranquillizers, sleeping tablets, blood pressure or weight-reducing tablets or tablets for the control of diabetes. They are also warned against the use of nasal decongestants and bronchial dilators.

Anticonvulsants

Carbamazepine (Tegretol) is now accepted as an anticonvulsant and an agent for the control of trigeminal neuralgia. It was claimed to be of benefit in migraine but a comparative trial in our own clinic was unable to substantiate this (Anthony and Lance, 1972).

Bradykinin antagonist

Methdilazine (Tacaryl, Dilosyn) is an N-substituted phenothiazine derivative with strong antihistamine and antibradykinin activity, and weak antiserotonin effects. When used as prophylactic therapy for migraine in the dose of 8 to 16 mg morning and night, it improved 41 per cent of patients, which was not significantly better than the placebo rate of 31 per cent (Lance, Anthony and Somerville, 1970). Drowsiness was a common side-effect.

Prostaglandin antagonists

Indomethacin (Indocid, Indocin)

When used in a large dose (150–200 mg daily) indomethacin is said to be beneficial in preventing migraine (Sicuteri, Michelacci and Anselmi, 1964). Large doses produce a high incidence of gastro-intestinal side-effects and may possibly be dangerous. A controlled trial of indomethacin, using the conventional dosage of 25 mg three times daily, showed that the drug was no more effective than placebo (Anthony and Lance, 1968). It is of interest that the daily use of indomethacin may cause a dull continuous headache.

Flufenamic acid (Flunalgin, Arlef)

The fenamates are said to inhibit the biosynthesis of prostaglandins and also to block certain actions of prostaglandins F and E. Vardi *et al.* (1976) have used flufenamic acid for the treatment of acute attacks of migraine in doses of 250 mg every two hours up to a maximum of 1 000 mg (8 tablets) with symptomatic relief in 195 of 200 treated attacks. Upper abdominal discomfort was experienced by 8 of 26 patients and another 2 patients had severe nausea and vomiting, one with melaena.

Aspirin

Aspirin reduces prostaglandin synthesis and also acts as a bradykinin antagonist although it is not known whether its action in relieving headache bears any relation to these properties. Trials of analgesic tablets compared with placebo have demonstrated that aspirin is superior to oral codeine, propoxyphene, phenacetin, pentazocine and mefenamic acid in the relief of malignant disease (Moertel, 1976) and this presumably applies to the pain of migraine, providing the aspirin can be adequately absorbed. Volans (1974) showed that 19 out of 42 migrainous patients had impaired absorption of aspirin at the time of migraine headache compared with normal controls and with their own absorption when headache-free. The Princess Margaret Migraine Clinic in London starts the treatment of an acute attack of migraine with an intramuscular injection of metoclopramide (Maxolon), 10 mg, to facilitate the absorption of ergotamine and aspirin given orally. The use of aspirin suppositories is also worthy of consideration.

Reserpine

Intermittent treatment with reserpine has been reported as being of use in the prophylaxis of migraine by Nattero and his colleagues (1976).

Levodopa

The use of L-Dopa for Parkinson's disease has been said to benefit migraine in those patients who suffer from both disorders, but there is still doubt about this.

Bromocriptine

Bromocriptine is a dopamine agonist which has been used in the management of Parkinson's disease and to suppress the secretion of growth hormone in acromegaly. It also suppresses prolactin secretion, and has been reported to reduce premenstrual symptoms and menstrual migraine when given in doses of 1 mg three times daily (Hockaday, Peet and Hockaday, 1976).

Heparin

On the basis that the basophil count in the blood of migrainous patients was lower than that of controls, that their basophils contained less heparin, and that they excreted less uroheparin than normal subjects, Thonnard-Neumann (1977) has used heparin in the treatment of migraine. He treated 27 patients with intravenous heparin and 33 patients with an aerosol form (2 500–5 000 units weekly) for an unspecified time and followed the patients for an average of 14 months after the course of treatment. He claimed that the migraine index (of frequency and severity of attacks) was reduced by 75 to 100 per cent in

18 of 27 patients treated by intravenous injections and 31 of 33 patients treated by the aerosol method, without any side-effects.

Isometheptene mucate

Isometheptene is an unsaturated aliphatic amine with sympathomimetic activity. Yuill, Swinburn and Liversedge (1972) compared the efficacy of this agent with that of ergotamine in treating 122 acute attacks of migraine. They considered that the intensity of headache and nausea was significantly less in the group treated with isometheptene although there was no difference in the duration of headache.

The extraordinary variety of drugs which have some effect on the migrainous process bears witness to the multifactorial nature of the disorder and leads to the conclusion that there is no one agent, or combination of agents, that is so effective that one can dispense with the rest. Fozard (1975) in a review of the pharmacology of drugs used in migraine commented that no single property of any drug in use could be unequivocally associated with clinical effectiveness.

TREATMENT OF THE ACUTE ATTACK OF MIGRAINE

Since the present concept of migraine headache is one of painful dilatation of cranial vessels, the object of handling an acute attack is to induce constriction of the scalp arteries, and to relieve pain and vomiting. Intravenous injection of serotonin or infusion of noradrenaline have been used experimentally to induce vasoconstriction with success in terminating migraine headache. These measures cause unpleasant side-effects and are not practicable for routine use. The agent accepted as safe and effective for some 50 years is ergotamine tartrate, which is considered to relieve the pain of migraine headache in about 70 per cent of patients. In one analysis of the response of 263 patients to treatment, ergotamine-containing preparations regularly relieved the headaches completely in 47 per cent and partially in 34 per cent (Selby and Lance, 1960). It is common for patients to state that their headaches last only 2 to 3 hours if they have access to ergotamine tartrate and for 12 to 24 hours if they do not. Some patients who vomit early in their attack are not helped by oral ergotamine tartrate but obtain rapid relief from the use of suppositories The intramuscular injection of metoclopramide (Maxolon), 10 mg, at the onset of an attack is used at the Princess Margaret Migraine Clinic, London, to reduce nausea and aid absorption of aspirin and ergotamine given orally. Ergotamine tartrate should be given at the first indication of a migraine attack, in adequate oral dosage (1–4 mg depending on the patient's weight and tolerance), in a form which is readily absorbed and acceptable to the patient. Nausea is a common side-effect and some patients complain of aching muscles. Vasoconstrictive phenomena are uncommon with the usual therapeutic doses of ergotamine tartrate but the appearance of signs of peripheral ischaemia may prevent its further use. Ergotamine tartrate has a slight oxytocic effect and should be used with caution in pregnancy. Habituation to ergot preparations may lead a migrainous patient to take daily medication, with a rebound headache developing every time the tablets are omitted. Supervised withdrawal in hospital may then become necessary.

There are now many preparations available, thus giving patients scope for experimentation to see which suits them best.

Ergotamine tartrate

(a) Coated tablets of ergotamine tartrate, 1 mg, (Femergin, Gynergen). One to three tablets should be swallowed at the onset of a migraine attack and repeated in half an hour if necessary. One tablet is usually sufficient as an initial dose for a child and two for most adults. If the attack is not aborted by the suggested two doses at half-hourly intervals, there is no point in taking more.

(b) Uncoated tablets of ergotamine tartrate, 1 mg, (Ergomar, Lingraine). These should be dissolved in the mouth and are then absorbed supposedly from the buccal mucosa. They were considered to act more rapidly than coated tablets by 40 per cent of our patients but some objected to their taste. The dosage schedule is the same for coated tablets.

(c) Aerosol form (Medihaler). A fine powder of ergotamine tartrate is available in pressure pack for inhalation. Instructions must be followed carefully so that the powder is inhaled deeply into the lungs. The device delivers 0·36 mg ergotamine at a time, and the inhalation can be repeated up to 6 times at intervals of 5 minutes.

(d) Injection. Ergotamine tartrate may be given by subcutaneous or intramuscular injection in doses of 0·25 to 0·5 mg.

Compounds containing ergotamine tartrate

Cafergot   Ergotamine tartrate, 1 mg, is combined with caffeine, 100 mg, in Cafergot tablets. One to two tablets are taken at the onset of migraine and repeated in half an hour if necessary.

Cafergot-PB suppositories Suppositories containing ergotamine tartrate, 2 mg, caffeine, 100 mg, belladonna alkaloids, 0·25 mg, and isobutyl allyl barbituric acid, 100 mg. One suppository is inserted rectally at the onset of migraine and this may be repeated in one hour if necessary. This form is particularly useful for those patients who become nauseated early in the attack when gastric absorption is impaired. Cramps in the thighs and drowsiness are not uncommon as side-effects.

Migral, Migril These tablets contain ergotamine tartrate, 2 mg, caffeine, 100 mg, with cyclizine, 50 mg, as an antiemetic. One tablet is taken at the onset of migraine and repeated in half an hour if necessary.

Ergodryl Ergotamine tartrate, 1 mg, caffeine, 100 mg, with diphenhydramine, 25 mg, as an antiemetic. One or two capsules are taken at the onset and repeated in half an hour if necessary.

There are a number of other combinations, containing different antiemetics, belladonna alkaloids or analgesics.

Isometheptene mucate

Capsules containing isometheptene, 65 mg, paracetamol, 325 mg, and dichloralphenazone, 100 mg (Midrid), have been reported as being effective in relieving acute attacks of migraine (Yuill, Swinburn and Liversedge, 1972).

Drugs to relieve pain and vomiting

Once a severe migraine headache is established, ergotamine tartrate is rarely of use and there is no alternative to symptomatic treatment with analgesics. The intravenous or intramuscular injection of diazepam (Valium), 10 mg, may be helpful as an antiemetic agent or one of the phenothiazine group such as prochlorperazine (Stemetil), 12·5 mg, or thiethylperazine dimaleate (Torecan), 10 mg, may be required to suppress vomiting. The latter group may occasionally give rise to dystonic reactions, so that it is worth having an ampoule of benztropine mesylate (Cogentin), 2 mg, available for intravenous injection should this occur.

PREVENTION OF FREQUENT ATTACKS BY INTERVAL MEDICATION

The prevention of migraine headache by continuous medication is a comparatively recent advance in the treatment of this disorder. When the frequency of migraine increases to two or more attacks each month, interval therapy must be considered. Before regular medication is started, it is important to consider whether one of the following factors could be responsible for the stepping up in intensity of the migrainous onslaught.

(1) Increased emotional or mental stress, such as a trap situation in the patient's private life or work.
(2) The onset of a depressive state.
(3) Increase in systemic blood pressure.
(4) The use of the contraceptive pill.
(5) Too frequent use of preparations containing ergotamine.

If the frequency of migraine attacks persists after attention to any of these factors which are relevant, it usually becomes necessary to prescribe a prophylactic drug to be taken two or three times daily in an endeavour to prevent the headaches completely or at least ameliorate their severity.

Sedatives and antidepressant drugs

Regular sedation is worth a trial in excitable children but is rarely effective in adults. Tranquillizing agents, such as diazepam (Valium), 2–5 mg, or chlordiazepoxide (Librium), 10 mg, three times daily are useful in those patients in whom nervous tension is playing a part in increasing the frequency of migraine attacks. Antidepressants, such as amitriptyline (Tryptanol, Tryptizol, Elavil, Laroxyl) 10–25 mg, or imipramine (Tofranil), 10–25 mg, three times daily may be of considerable indirect benefit. It is probable that anticonvulsant and conventional antihistamine drugs have no advantage over other sedatives in the treatment of migraine. It must be remembered that fluctuations occur in the natural history of migraine, and the psychological boost of any new treatment will give a certain placebo response, amounting to 20 to 30 per cent of patients improved.

Ergotamine tartrate and related preparations

The use of ergotamine tartrate for prophylaxis is limited by the relatively short duration of its vasoconstrictor action, but some patients find they can prevent a nocturnal or early morning attack of migraine by taking 1 to 2 mg on retiring. Barrie, *et al.*

(1968) undertook a controlled trial of ergotamine tartrate, 0·5 or 1·0 mg daily, ergometrine maleate, 1·0 or 2·0 mg daily, and methysergide maleate (Deseril, Sansert), 3.0 or 6.0 mg daily in 105 outpatients with frequent migraine attacks. They concluded that methysergide was marginally more effective than the other drugs but produced more side-effects.

A preparation containing phenobarbitone, 20 mg, ergotamine tartrate, 0·3 mg, and belladonna alkaloids, 0·1 mg (Bellergal), when given as one tablet three times daily, is more effective than simple sedation and gives improvement in about 35 per cent of patients (Curran and Lance, 1964). This is a useful medication for children, one tablet each night often being sufficient to reduce substantially the frequency of migraine headache.

Dihydroergotamine (DHE) has been used for many years as a prophylactic agent for migraine, particularly in Europe, but the author is not aware of any comparative assessment of its merits.

Interval therapy in common use

Any patient experiencing two or more attacks each month which are not responsive to ergotamine or simple analgesics warrants a thorough trial of interval therapy. My own practice is to start with those agents which are less effective but have less side-effects than methysergide or the MAO inhibitors.

Pizotifen (Sandomigran), 0·5 mg, can be given as one tablet morning and night at first, the dose being increased to one tablet three times daily if the patient is not drowsy. If the response to this is satisfactory, the patient can be maintained on it for years if necessary as no long-term side-effects have been described. If there is no improvement after one month, propranolol (Inderal) 40-mg tabs can be prescribed, starting with one-half tablet three times daily and increasing to one or even two tablets three times daily if the drug is tolerated well. It should not be used in patients prone to bronchospasms or postural hypotension. Conversely, it is a particularly useful drug in migrainous patients who are hypertensive. Clonidine also finds a place in patients with the combination of migraine and hypertension.

Should the patient show inadequate improvement after these opening shots have been fired, a trial of methysergide is warranted. Much has been written about the side-effects of methysergide but if used cautiously it is not hazardous, and it is certainly the most effective preparation at present available for the control of migraine. It is recommended that treatment be ceased for one month after every four months to minimize the possibility of fibrotic side-effects, which are rare in any event even with long-term medication.

It is advisable to give a trial dose of 1 mg and then to increase the dose at daily intervals from 1 mg twice daily up to 2 mg three times daily if necessary. The tablets are best taken after meals to minimize epigastric discomfort. Dosage and timing can be adjusted to suit the requirements of each particular patient. A patient who is invariably awakened at 3 a.m. by an attack may be controlled by nocturnal medication only. A woman whose attacks are more frequent with menstruation may require increased dosage at that time.

Patients who become virtually free of headache while taking 6 mg daily may slowly reduce the dose to a minimum which will maintain control. When a patient who has been maintained on methysergide ceases treatment for one month every four, it is advisable to withdraw the drug slowly in order to prevent a severe 'rebound headache'. Methysergide does not appear to have any curative effect and must be continued as long as the tendency to headache persists.

Methysergide is not effective for the treatment of the acute attack in most instances, although some patients whose frequency of headache has diminished under treatment may find that some episodes can be aborted by taking their dose of methysergide at the first symptom of an attack. Ergotamine preparations may be used for the acute attack in the usual way if some headaches occur while the patient is under treatment with methysergide, and they are then often more effective than before.

If the patient proves resistant to pizotifen, propranolol and methysergide, my own practice is to prescribe the MAO inhibitor phenelzine (Nardil), 15 mg twice daily, increasing to three or four tablets daily if necessary and if the patient is not overstimulated. Those patients who have difficulty in sleeping while taking phenelzine may have to limit themselves to one tablet in the morning and one at noon. Providing the restrictions on diet and drug intake mentioned earlier in this chapter are observed, the treatment appears to be completely safe and the results are usually satisfactory. I have not had any patient suffer a hypertensive crisis but some have the reverse problem of postural hypotension. Some male patients mention that it takes longer to achieve orgasm while taking phenelzine but there are few complaints about this side-effect.

There remain some patients who continue to have their migraine attacks unabated by all forms of pharmacotherapy. These patients may benefit from admission to hospital to isolate them from their normal environment, the withdrawal of all medication, and full attention being paid to psychological management and relaxation training. The patient with 'status migrainosus' (daily severe headaches persisting in spite of hospital admission) may benefit from an intravenous infusion of procaine or Xylocaine as described for the treatment of postherpetic neuralgia, or may be given a short course of prednisone 60 mg daily.

General conclusions about the drug treatment of migraine

When attacks are infrequent, it is pointless to prescribe interval medication. If the patient is able to anticipate when the next episode is coming because of the association with a precipitating factor, such as menstruation, or because of some sensation, such as an intense feeling of well-being, which regularly precedes an attack, then treatment may be planned accordingly. Ergotamine tartrate may be given the night before the migraine headache is anticipated, or methysergide may be started 24 hours before if there is sufficient warning.

The treatment of the acute attack still relies on an adequate dose of ergotamine tartrate given in the form most acceptable to the patient, usually as a tablet or suppository. The suppository is particularly useful in patients who vomit early in the headache and have no time to absorb oral medication.

In patients who are subject to two migraine headaches or more each month, a thorough trial of interval treatment should be given, much in the same way as anticonvulsants are used in epilepsy, with the aim of eliminating the attacks completely.

Migraine is a difficult problem to treat but we can never say to a patient that his illness cannot be helped until we have tried conscientiously all kinds of medicines 'Cephalics, Hysterical, all famous Specificks'. Otherwise, as Willis foretold, our patients will turn to the unlearned, quacks and old women.

REFERENCES

Aellig, W.H. and Berde, B. (1969). Ergot compounds and vascular resistance. *Br. J. Pharmac.* **36**, 561

Anderson, J.A.D.. Basker, M.A. and Dalton, R. (1975). Migraine and hypnotherapy. *Int. J. clin. exp. Hypnosis.* **23**, 48

Anthony, M. and Lance, J.W. (1968). Indomethacin in migraine. *Med. J. Aust.* **1**, 56

Anthony, M. and Lance, J.W. (1969). Monoamine oxidase inhibition in the treatment of migraine. *Archs Neurol.* **21**, 263

Anthony, M. and Lance, J. W. (1972). A comparative trial of prindolol, clonidine and carbamazepine in the interval therapy of migraine. *Med. J. Aust.* **1**, 1343

Barrie, M.A., Carpenter, M.E., Carroll, J.D., Knawlson, P.A., Neylan, C., Ross, O.,

Rowsell, A.R. and Wilkinson, M.I.P. (1971). The use of clonidine (ST155) in migraine and the problems encountered in a multicentric trial. In *Proceedings of the International Headache Symposium, Elsinore, Denmark* p. 23. Basle: Sandoz

Barrie, M.A., Fox, W.R., Weatherall, M. and Wilkinson, M.I.P. (1968). Analysis of symptoms of patients with headaches and their response to treatment with ergot derivatives. *Q. J. Med.* **37**, 319

Benson, H., Klemchuk, H.P. and Graham, J.R. (1974). The usefulness of the relaxation response in the therapy of headache. *Headache* **14**, 49

Berde, B. (1972). Recent progress in the elucidation of the mechanism of action of ergot compounds used in migraine therapy. *Med. J. Aust.* **2**, 15 (Suppl.)

Bianchine, J.R. and Eade, N.R. (1967). The effect of 5-hydroxytryptamine on the cotton pellet local inflammatory response in the rat. *J. exp. Med.* **125**, 501

Blumenthal, L.S. and Fuchs, M. (1963). Current therapy for headache. *Sth med. J., Nashville* **56**, 503

Carroll, P.R., Ebeling, P.W. and Glover, W.E. (1974). The responses of the human temporal and rabbit ear artery to 5-hydroxytryptamine and some of its antagonists. *Aust. J. exp. Biol. med. Sci.* **52**, 813

Couch, J.R., Ziegler, D.K. and Hassanein, R. (1976). Amitriptyline in the prophylaxis of migraine. Effectiveness and relationship of antimigraine and antidepressant drugs. *Neurology* **26**, 121

Cook, N. (1973) Cryosurgery of migraine. *Headache* **12**, 143

Curran, D.A. Hinterberger, H. and Lance, J.W. (1967). Methysergide. *Res. clin. Stud. Headache* **1**, 74

Curran, D.A. and Lance, J.W. (1964). Clinical trial of methysergide and other preparations in the management of migraine. *J. Neurol. Neurosurg. Psychiat.* **27**, 463

Cyriax, J. (1962). *Text-book of Orthopaedic Medicine*, Vol. 1, p.193. London: Cassell

Dalessio, D.J., Camp, W.A., Goodell, H. and Wolff, H.G. (1961). Studies on headache. The mode of action of UML-491 and its relevance to the nature of vascular headache of the migraine type. *Archs Neurol.* **4**, 235

Diamond, S. and Medina, J.L. (1976). Double-blind study of propranolol for migraine prophylaxis. *Headache* **16**, 24

Edmeads, J., Hachinski, V.C. and Norris, J.W. (1976). Ergotamine and the cerebral circulation. *Hemicrania* **7**, 6

Ekbom, K. (1975). Adrenergic beta-receptor blockers. In *Vasoactive Substances Relevant to Migraine.* Ed. S. Diamond, D.J. Dalessio, J.R. Graham and J.L. Medina. p. 19. Springfield, Illinois: Thomas

Forssman, B., Henriksson, K-G., Johannson, V., Lindvall, L. and Lundin, H-₵. (1976). Propranolol for migraine prophylaxis. *Headache* **16**, 238

Fozard, J. (1975). Pharmacology of drugs used in migraine. *J. Pharm. Pharmac.* **27**, 297

Friedman, A.P. (1970). The (Infinite) variety of migraine. In *Background to Migraine*, Third British Migraine Symposium, p. 165. London: Heinemann.

Gomersall, J.D. and Stuart, A. (1973). Amitriptyline in migraine prophylaxis. Changes in pattern of attacks during a controlled clinical trial. *J. Neurol. Neurosurg. Psychiat.* **36**, 684

Graham, J.R. (1967). Cardiac and pulmonary fibrosis during methysergide therapy for headache. *Am. J. med. Sci.* **254**, 23

Hockaday, J.M., Peet, K.M.S., and Hockaday, T.D.R. (1976). Bromocriptine in migraine. *Headache* **16**, 109

206 The Treatment of Migraine

Hudgson, P., Foster, J.B. and Newell, D.J. (1967). Controlled trial of Demigran in the prophylaxis of migraine. *Br. med. J.* **1**, 91
Kajdos, V. (1975). The acupuncture treatment of headaches. *Am. J. Acupuncture* **3**, 34
Koppman, J.W., McDonald, R.D. and Kunzel, M.G. (1974). Voluntary regulation of temporal artery diameter by migraine patients. *Headache* **14**, 133
Lance, J.W., Anthony, M. and Somerville, B. (1970). Comparative trial of serotonin antagonists in the management of migraine. *Br. med. J.* **2**, 327
Lance, J.W., Fine, R.D. and Curran, D.A. (1963). An evaluation of methysergide in the prevention of migraine and other vascular headaches. *Med. J. Aust.* **1**, 814
Lewis, C.T., Molland, E.A., Marshall, V.R., Tresidder, G.C. and Blandy, J.P. (1975). Analgesic abuse, ureteric obstruction, and retroperitoneal fibrosis. *Br. med. J.* **2**, 76
Lundberg, P.O. (1962). Migraine prophylaxis with progestogens. *Acta endocr. Copenh.* **40**, (Suppl. 68), 5
Medina, J.L., Diamond, S. and Franklin, M.A. (1976). Biofeedback therapy for migraine. *Headache* **16**, 115
Meier, J. and Schreier, E. (1976). Human plasma levels of some anti-migraine drugs. *Headache* **16**, 96
Mitchell, K.R. and Mitchell, D.M. (1971). Migraine: an exploratory treatment application of programmed behaviour therapy techniques. *J. psychosom. Res.* **15**, 137
Mitchell, K.R. and White, R.G. (1976). The control of migraine headache by behavioural self-management: a controlled case study. *Headache* **16**, 178
Moertel, C.G. (1976). Relief of pain with oral medications. *Aust. N.Z. Jl Med.* **6**, (Suppl. 1), 1
Mylecharane, E.J., Duckworth, J.W., Lord, G.D.A. and Lance, J.W. (1977). Effects of low doses of clonidine in anaesthetized monkeys. *Proc. Aust. physiol. pharmac. Soc.* **8**, 42P
Mylecharane, E.J., Spira, P.J., Misbach, J. Duckworth, J.W. and Lance, J.W. (1977). Effects of methysergide, pizotifen and ergotamine in the monkey cranial circulation. *Europ. J. Pharmacol.* In press
Nattero, G., Lisino, F., Brandi, G., Gastaldi, L. and Genefke, I.K. (1976). Reserpine for migraine prophylaxis. *Headache* **15**, 279
Price, K.P. and Tursky, B. (1976). Vascular reactivity of migraineurs and non-migraineurs: a comparison of responses to self-control procedures. *Headache* **16**, 210
Rompel, H. and Bauermeister, P.W. (1970). Aetiology of migraine and prevention with carbamazepine (Tegretol): results of a double-blind crossover study. *S. Afr. Gr. med. J.* **44**, 75
Ryan, R.E. and Robert, R.E., Jr. (1975). Clonidine – its use in migraine therapy. *Headache* **14**, 191
Sargent, J.D., Green, E.E. and Walters, E.D. (1972). The use of autogenic feedback training in a pilot study of migraine and tension headaches. *Headache* **12**, 120
Saxena, P.R. (1972). The effect of antimigraine drugs on the vascular responses of 5-hydroxytryptamine and related biogenic substances on the external carotid bed of dogs: possible pharmacological implications to their antimigraine action. *Headache* **12**, 44
Selby, G. and Lance, J.W. (1960). Observations on 500 cases of migraine and allied vascular headache. *J. Neurol. Neurosurg. Psychiat.* **23**, 23

Shafar, J., and Tallett, E.R. (1972). Evaluation of clonidine in prophylaxis of migraine. *Lancet* **1**, 403

Shaw, D.A. and Saunders, M. (1972). A double-blind comparison of Dixarit and placebo. In *The Migraine Headache and Dixarit* p. 54. Bracknell, Berkshire: Boehringer Ingelheim

Sicuteri, F., Michelacci, S. and Anselmi, B. (1964). Individuazione della proprieta vasoattive ed antiemicraniche dell' indomethacin, nuovo antiflogistico di derivazione indolica. *Settim. med.* **52**, 335

Speight, T.M. and Avery, G.S. (1972). Pizotifen (BC105): a review of its pharmacological properties and its therapeutic efficacy in vascular headache. *Drugs* **3**, 153

Spira, P.J., Mylecharane, E.J. and Lance, J.W. (1976). The effects of humoral agents and antimigraine drugs on the cranial circulation of the monkey. *Res. clin. Stud. Headache* **4**, 37

Stensrud, P. and Sjaastad, O. (1976a). Short-term clinical trial of propranolol in racemic form (Inderal), d-propranolol and placebo in migraine. *Acta neurol. scand.* **53**, 229

Stensrud, P. and Sjaastad, O. (1976b). Clonidine (Catapresan) – double-blind study after long-term treatment with the drug in migraine. *Acta neurol. scand.* **53**, 233

Thonnard-Neumann, E. (1977). Migraine therapy with heparin: pathophysiologic basis. *Headache* **16**, 284

Vardi, Y., Rabey, I.M., Streifler, M., Schwartz, A., Lindner, H.R. and Zor, U. (1976). Migraine attacks. Alleviation by an inhibitor of prostaglandin synthesis and action. *Neurology* **26**, 447

Volans, G.N. (1974). Absorption of effervescent aspirin during migraine. *Br. med. J.* **2**, 265

Warner, G. and Lance, J.W. (1975). Relaxation therapy in migraine and tension headache. *Med. J. Aust.* **1**, 298

Weber, R.B. and Reinmuth, O.M. (1971). The treatment of migraine with propranolol. *Neurology* **21**, 404

Widerøe, T-E and Vigander, T. (1974). Propranolol in the treatment of migraine. *Br. med. J.* **1**, 699

Wolff, H.G. (1963). *Headache and Other Head Pain*. London/New York: Oxford University Press.

Yuill, G.M. Swinburn, W.R. and Liversedge, L.A. (1972). A double-blind crossover trial of isometheptene mucate compound and ergotamine in migraine. *Br. J. clin. Pract.* **26**, 76

Zaimis, E. and Hanington, E. (1969). A possible pharmacological approach to migraine. *Lancet* **2**, 298

Thirteen
Cluster Headache (Migrainous Neuralgia)

Periodic migrainous neuralgia or cluster headache may be defined as a severe unilateral head or facial pain, which lasts for minutes or hours, associated commonly with ipsilateral lacrimation and blockage of the nostril, usually recurring once or more daily for a period of weeks or months. The term cluster headache derives from the tendency for the pain to appear in bouts, separated by intervals of complete freedom (Kunkle *et al.*, 1954).

In 1840, Romberg described as 'ciliary neuralgia' recurrent pain in the eye, which was generally confined to one side and associated with photophobia. 'The pupil is contracted. The pain not infrequently extends over the head and face. The eye generally weeps and becomes red. These symptoms occur in paroxysms of a uniform or irregular character, and isolated or combined with facial neuralgia and hemicrania.' Romberg considered that scrofula was the main cause of ciliary neuralgia but that it was also brought on by discharges, especially seminal emissions. The condition was first recorded in the English medical literature by Harris in 1926 as ciliary (migrainous) neuralgia and this description was later elaborated (Harris, 1936).

The uncertainty about the nature and aetiology of this disorder is reflected by other names which have been used to describe similar syndromes over the past century such as red migraine, erythroprosopalgia, erythromelalgia of the head, syndrome of hemicephalic vasodilation of sympathetic origin, autonomic faciocephalalgia, greater superficial petrosal neuralgia and histamine cephalalgia (Ekbom, 1970; Friedman and Mikropoulos, 1958; Robinson, 1958; Sutherland and Eadie, 1972). Symonds (1956) used the non-committal title of 'a particular variety of

208

headache'. Sphenopalatine neurosis (Sluder, 1910) and vidian neuralgia (Vail, 1932) were described as affecting mostly female patients and appear more akin to lower half headache, now known as facial migraine, than to the syndrome under discussion.

The nature of the attack and pattern of recurrence of this syndrome are so characteristic that it can readily be distinguished from migraine and trigeminal neuralgia. In spite of this the majority of patients are referred to neurological clinics with the provisional diagnosis of one or the other of these disorders, and the condition is usually referred to in the British literature as 'migrainous neuralgia'.

Cluster headache is considerably less common than migraine. Friedman diagnosed 237 cases of cluster headache and 2 667 migrainous patients over a 9-year period. In published series cluster headache varies in incidence from 2 to 9 per cent of that of migraine (Ekbom, 1970).

CLINICAL FEATURES

Sex incidence

Cluster headache is a notable exception to feminine dominance of the problem of chronic headache. Most series favour males in the ratio of 3–6:1. Of 60 of our patients only 8 were female. The male:female ratio was thus 6·5:1;

Age of onset

The illness begins in the second and third decades of life in the majority of patients (*Figure 13.1*). In our series of 60 patients (Lance and Anthony, 1971), 15 (25 per cent) started to have attacks between the ages of 16 and 20 years and 35 (68 per cent) between 11 and 30 years. One patient became subject to isolated episodes of retro-orbital pain and lacrimation at the age of 8 years, which recurred twice each year until typical bouts occurred in his second decade. The latest age of onset was 62 years.

Site of pain

The pain of cluster headache is unilateral, almost always affecting the same side of the head in each bout, although there have been cases reported in which it has changed sides in different bouts. In 32 of our

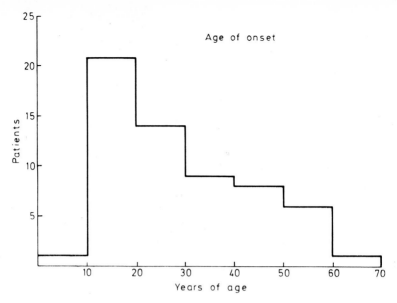

Figure 13.1. The age of onset of cluster headache in 60 patients (from Lance and Anthony, 1971)

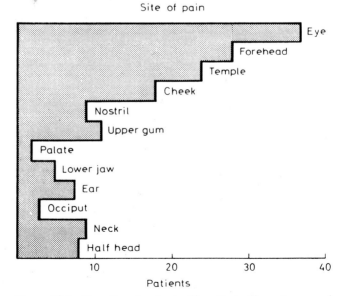

Figure 13.2. The site of pain in 60 patients (from Lance and Anthony, 1971)

60 patients, the attacks were exclusively right-sided, in 23 left-sided and in 5 the side affected varied from bout to bout or on different days in the same bout. The pain is felt deeply in and around the eye by about 60 per cent of patients (*Figure 13.2*). It commonly radiates to the supra-orbital region, temple, maxilla and upper gum on the same side of the face. In some patients the ipsilateral nostril aches and burns, and a few complain of aching in the roof of the mouth. In other patients, the lower gum, jaw or chin are also involved. The pain may spread to the ear, the neck or 'the entire half of the head'.

Quality of pain

The pain of cluster headache is peculiarly distressing. It may be throbbing or pulsating on occasions but the majority describe the pain as constant and severe. Common adjectives used to describe it are burning, boring, piercing, tearing and screwing. One patient stated that it was like a blunt knife being pushed in and turned. Two of our patients said that a dull background pain persisted in the temple or upper jaw between attacks, and 4 patients mentioned a dull ache preceding a bout by some hours or days. Three patients said that they had sometimes experienced sudden jabs of pain in the affected areas at the time of the headache. We have had experience of 3 patients whose cluster headaches were associated with tic douloureux. A summary of a case history is presented here because of its relevance to a possible neural mechanism for the syndrome.

CASE REPORT

Cluster headache associated with tic douloureux:
A man aged 46 years was well until the age of 42 when he first developed transient shooting, stabbing pains in the inner side of the right lower gum and the adjacent right side of the tongue, which were brought on by movements of the tongue. The pain was severe and initially recurred as single jabs, then as repeated jabs intermittently through the day. After 2 weeks the pain spread to involve the upper gum, and each stab radiated to the midline of the upper and lower jaw. After 3 months each pain seemed to flash up to the right temple and in front of the right temporomandibular joint 'as a single hit'.
Two months later he had his first attack of headache which followed a bad episode of his jabbing pain. On this occasion, pain remained in the right temple for half an hour. The right eye watered,

the right nostril ached and discharged a clear fluid. This more prolonged pain lasted for 30 minutes and returned 3 times daily for
some weeks. After 1 month the pain radiated up to the vertex and
persisted for 30 to 90 minutes, recurring 2 to 3 times daily. After 5
days this variety of pain disappeared but the jabbing pain continued.
The jabbing pains were precipitated by swallowing, talking or
touching the right lower lip and were stopped by taking carbamazepine, 400 mg, three times daily.

The pain in the temple radiating up to the vertex disappeared for
2 months at a time, would return for 5 days, then again vanish, and
recurred in this pattern for 3 years. When the tic-like pain was controlled by carbamazepine, the cluster headache ceased. The tic-like
pain, but not the cluster type of pain, recurred after 12 months of
treatment with carbamazepine. The second and third divisions of the
trigeminal nerve were then sectioned intracranially with complete
relief of pain. No abnormality was seen in the Gasserian ganglion or
trigeminal nerve at operation.

A similar association has been reported previously by others
(Sutherland and Eadie, 1972).

Periodicity of bouts

Cluster headache is so called because of its tendency to recur in bouts
or clusters, although about one-fifth of patients with the characteristic
pain and accompaniments have a pattern of recurrence which resembles
that of migraine without any long periods of freedom. These are desig-
nated 'non-cluster' in *Figure 13.3* and are sometimes called chronic

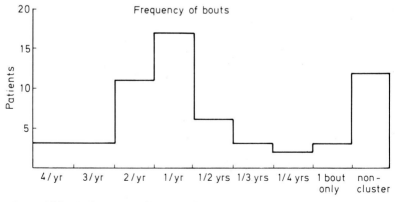

Figure 13.3. The frequency of bouts in 60 patients (from Lance and Anthony, 1971)

cluster headache. Four of our patients were subject to attacks of pain from 1 to 4 times a week without ever having suffered a bout of regular daily episodes. The other 8 of our non-cluster or chronic cluster headache patients had started in this manner but the frequency had increased until they were experiencing from 1 to 5 attacks daily. The remaining patients of our series were subject to bouts with sufficient regularity to enable them to be classified in *Figure 13.3*. Most patients suffered 1 or 2 bouts each year.

The periodicity of bouts did not depend consistently upon the time of year. Of those who considered that their bouts had a seasonal incidence, 5 stated that they recurred in spring, 6 in summer, 6 in autumn and 7 in winter.

Duration of bouts

The usual length of each bout is shown in *Figure 13.4*, from 4 to 8 weeks being the most common. It should be noted that within the 'non-cluster' category are included some patients who had been experiencing

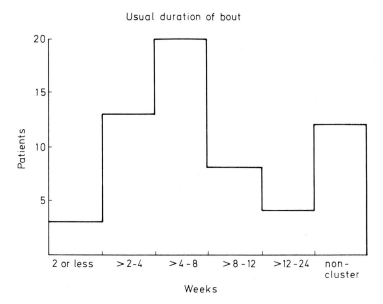

Figure 13.4. The usual duration of each bout in 60 patients (from Lance and Anthony, 1971)

daily attacks for 12 months without any indication of such a prolonged 'bout' ending.

Daily frequency of attacks during a bout

The usual number of attacks daily is from 1 to 3 as shown in *Figure 13.5* but the maximum may be 8 or more. The 4 of our patients who had never experienced headaches every day are excluded from *Figure13.5*. Sjaastad and Dale (1974) described 2 patients who experienced as many as 12 to 18 attacks in 24 hours.

Of our 60 patients, 52 stated that their attacks were liable to recur at a particular time of the day or night, 32 mentioned 'night time', 9 specifically from 10 p.m. to 2 a.m., and 13 from 2 a.m. to 6 a.m.

Duration of attacks

Each particular episode usually starts suddenly, lasts for 10 minutes to 2 hours (*Figure 13.6*) and may end abruptly or fade away more slowly.

Associated features (Table 13.1)

Lacrimation from the eye on the affected side is the most common symptom and occasionally lacrimation is bilateral. The conjunctiva is often injected on the side of the headache. Drooping of the ipsilateral eyelid and miosis occur in about one-third of patients and may, rarely, persist between attacks (*see Figure 5.1*). Some complain of excessive bilateral sweating during attacks, including patients with ptosis and miosis, indicating that the ocular sympathetic nerve supply is involved discretely. Blurred vision may be noticed in the ipsilateral eye, which cannot be attributed to excessive lacrimation since some do not have this symptom.

The nostril is often blocked or running on one or both sides. A running nostril cannot be explained by lacrimation in all cases since it is not always associated with a weeping eye.

Gastro-intestinal disturbances are less common than in migraine but about one-half the patients feel nauseated and may vomit. Two of our patients were certain that nausea preceded the onset of facial pain on each occasion.

Vascular phenomena are particularly interesting. The superficial temporal artery on the affected side may become prominent, more

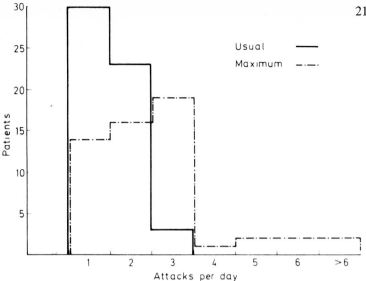

Figure 13.5. The number of attacks experienced per day. Continuous line, usual frequency; interrupted line, maximum frequency for each patient (from Lance and Anthony, 1971)

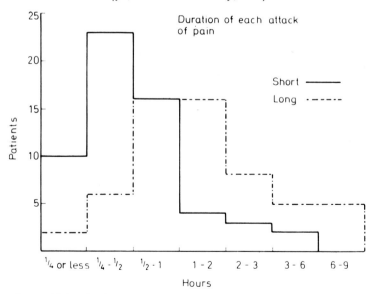

Figure 13.6. The duration of the attacks of pain. Continuous line, the shortest attacks; interrupted line, the longest attack experienced by each patient (from Lance and Anthony, 1971)

TABLE 13.1
Associated features in 60 patients (Lance and Anthony, 1971)

Ocular

lacrimation { unilateral		49
{ bilateral		3
conjunctival injection		27
partial Horner's syndrome		19
photophobia		12
blurred vision		5

Nasal

blocked nostril { unilateral		28
{ bilateral		4
running nostril { unilateral		9
{ bilateral		1
epistaxis		1

Gastro-intestinal

anorexia		2
nausea		26
vomiting { occasionally		9
{ regularly		8
diarrhoea		2

Vascular

flushing of face	12
pallor of face	2
prominent, tender temporal artery	10
prominent veins in forehead	2
puffiness around eyes	6
lumps in mouth	2
cold hands and feet	1
polyuria	4

Neurological

hyperalgesia of scalp and face	10
itching behind eye (preceding headache)	2
flashing lights in front of eyes	1
spots in front of eyes	1
vertigo and mild ataxia	4
mental confusion	1
unilateral carpal spasm	1

than usually pulsatile, and tender to touch; superficial veins may dilate. Four of our patients stated that their pain was relieved by compressing the temporal artery, although one emphasized that pain still persisted deep to the eye. Facial flushing is more common than pallor and was the origin of the old term 'red migraine'.

Hyperalgesia of the face and scalp is common and can be extreme in some cases so that the patient cannot bear to touch the affected areas. Two of our patients had noticed an itching sensation behind the eye, one immediately preceding pain in the eye and the other for some weeks before a bout began.

Focal neurological symptoms or signs, of the type which are common in migraine, are unusual in cluster headache. One of our patients mentioned occasional 'spots before the eyes' and another described 'little flashing lights in front of the eyes' during the headache. Four described a feeling of dizziness, giddiness, or a 'rising feeling in the head' associated with impaired balance at the time of the attack. One patient had experienced a tonic seizure of the left arm on three occasions associated with a pain in the right eye and temple. The left hand assumed the position of carpal spasm for a period of minutes. Sutherland and Eadie (1972) reported a patient who was subject to scintillating scotomata before cluster headache, 2 patients with paraesthesiae on the side of the body opposite to the head pain, and 1 patient with twitching of the contralateral foot.

Precipitating factors

The only trigger factor which is consistently mentioned by patients is the taking of alcoholic drinks and this is only operative during a susceptible period, that is to say, during a bout. Other vasodilator substances have been used experimentally to precipitate an attack. One of our patients who used carbon tetrachloride as a solvent in his daily work commented that inhalation of the fumes would induce an attack as readily as alcohol. Other factors mentioned by patients are stress, attacks of hay fever, heat, changes in weather, glare, missing a meal or sleeping late in the mornings.

Relieving factors

Some patients can find some ease from their pain by pressing on the superficial temporal arteries, by the application of heat, or by pacing up and down with their hand clasped over one eye.

PAST HISTORY

There is nothing very remarkable in the past health of patients with cluster headache and no convincing association with migraine or allergic disorders.

Migraine

Four of our 60 patients had been subject to frequent vomiting attacks in childhood and there was a history of migraine in 4 patients, 1 of whom continued to have occasional migraine headaches between bouts of cluster headache.

Allergy

Of 60 patients, 9 had suffered from allergic disorders, 2 from hives, 2 from asthma, 4 from hay fever and 1 from both asthma and hay fever. Two patients were of particular interest in that bouts of cluster headache regularly followed 2 to 4 weeks after episodes of hay fever. One of these patients stated that his hay fever was becoming milder each year but that his bouts of cluster headache were becoming longer and more severe. Allergy tests were performed in 4 patients, 1 of whom had a history of hives, but no positive skin test was obtained.

Trauma

Eight of our 60 patients had experienced a head injury, and in 4 the site of injury could conceivably be relevant to the ensuing cluster headache. One patient had required extensive plastic surgery for facial and scalp lacerations following a car accident and left-sided cluster headache started 21 months after injury. The second had gravel embedded in the right temple from a road accident at the age of 17 years and cluster headaches involving the right temple and right side of the face began 7 years later. The third patient developed right frontotemporal cluster headache 30 years after a shotgun injury to the forehead, in which fragmented pellets were still embedded. The fourth patient experienced a blow on the forehead at the age of 22 years, following which he was subject to a dull right-sided headache for 3 years. Eight years after the injury, right-sided cluster headaches developed, involving the right forehead and right side of the face.

Other illnesses of possible relevance

Disorders worthy of note in our series were meningitis 7 years before the onset of cluster headache, right-sided stapedectomy 6 months before the onset of right-sided cluster headache, excessive lacrimation of the right eye without obvious ocular cause for 3 years before bouts of pain in the right eye started, and loss of pinprick and temperature sensation over the right side of the neck and right arm in a man of 52, 6 years before right-sided cluster headache began. One female patient suffered from chronic lymphatic leukaemia, and one male patient had required treatment for a depressive state.

FAMILY HISTORY

Of our 60 patients, 13 had a family history of migraine affecting a parent or sibling. None had any member of the family afflicted by cluster headache. The incidence of migraine in parents and siblings (22 per cent in our series) is not significantly greater than that of patients with tension headache (18 per cent) and much less than that of typical migrainous patients (45 per cent) (Lance and Anthony, 1966). Ekbom (1970) found a family history of migraine in 16 per cent of patients with cluster headache compared with 65 per cent of migrainous patients. It is rare to find other examples of cluster headache in the family history. Examples have been cited by Bickerstaff (1959). Nieman and Hurwitz (1961), Balla and Walton (1964), Sutherland and Eadie (1972), and Ekbom (1970).

PATHOPHYSIOLOGY

IS THIS SYNDROME A VARIANT OF MIGRAINE?

The common denominator of both migraine and cluster headache is dilatation of the extracranial arteries, although this is strictly unilateral in cluster headache and tends to become bilateral in migraine. The internal carotid artery is also involved in most patients with cluster headache as judged by the frequency of retro-orbital pain and of paralysis of the ocular sympathetic supply, which most authorities agree is caused by compression of the sympathetic plexus in the carotid canal by distension of the wall of the internal carotid artery (Kunkle and Anderson, 1961; Nieman and Hurwitz, 1961). The localization of the lesion in the sympathetic pathway is aided by the sparing of facial sweating, which is mediated by the sympathetic plexus surrounding extracranial vessels.

Kunkle *et al.* (1954) injected normal saline intrathecally under pressure without benefit in 2 patients, but these patients had responded to ergotamine tartrate, suggesting that arterial vasodilatation was mainly extracranial in their cases. The dual source of pain in cluster headache, intracranial and extracranial, is illustrated by one of our patients who found that he could relieve the pain in his temple by compressing his dilated superficial temporal artery, but that some pain persisted, felt deeply behind the eye. Ekbom and Greitz (1970) reported vascular changes demonstrated by angiography during an episode of cluster headache. At the height of the attack, the internal carotid artery showed localized narrowing after emerging from the carotid canal; this was attributed to oedema or spasm and persisted after pain had ceased. In contrast, the ophthalmic artery was dilated during the attack.

The importance of vascular dilatation in cluster headache is emphasized by the ease with which headaches may be triggered during a bout by vasodilators such as alcohol, histamine (Horton, MacLean and Craig, 1939) and nitroglycerin (Ekbom, 1970) and their prevention by the prophylactic use of ergotamine tartrate (Symonds, 1956) or regular medication with methysergide (Curran, Hinterberger and Lance, 1967).

One important difference between the vascular changes of migraine and cluster headache is that the majority of patients become pale in migraine because of constriction of cutaneous capillaries, whereas this is uncommon in cluster headache (2 out of 60 in our series). On the contrary, 12 of our patients (20 per cent) noticed flushing of face. Horton, MacLean and Craig (1939) noted that skin temperatures were 1 to 3 degC higher on the side of the headache. Recent thermographic studies demonstrated an increase of skin temperature over the painful area in only 3 of the 5 patients studied (Plate 1). Two of these patients showed a 'cold spot' over the eye on the affected side in the early phase of headache (Plate 1) which is very similar to the cold area observed on the forehead of patients with stenosis or occlusion of the internal carotid artery because of inadequate filling of the terminal branches of the ophthalmic artery which supply the skin of the forehead. The 'cold spots' which have been noted on the forehead of patients with cluster headache by Wood and Friedman (1976) are in the same distribution and can be seen in Plate 1h. Broch et al. (1970) have reported that blood-flow in the internal carotid artery was unaltered in 3 patients during cluster headache, so that the mechanism of the cool forehead cannot be explained by constriction of the lumen of the carotid artery. Observations of the corneal indentation pulse pattern in cluster headache suggests that the intra-ocular vascular bed is dilated (Hørven, Nornes and Sjaastad, 1972). It is possible that flow in the ophthalmic artery reverses during the early stages of cluster headache or that its cutaneous branches are constricted. At a later stage of the headache, the temperature of the forehead and affected areas increases in most patients. The frequency of conjunctival injection and nasal blockage in cluster headache supports the view that facial and scalp capillaries dilate. This may be associated with oedema, causing swelling of the periorbital region or buccal mucosa.

Visual disturbance, such as zig-zags of light (fortification spectra, teichopsia) or unformed flashes of light (photopsia) are very common in migraine, affecting 30 to 40 per cent of patients before or during the headache, but are very rare in cluster headache.

Considering the vascular phenomena of migraine and cluster headache, the following tentative comparison may be drawn. In migraine, vessels supplying the cerebral cortex often constrict, some large intracranial arteries may dilate, extracranial arteries dilate and scalp and facial capillaries usually constrict. In cluster headache, the ophthalmic artery, extracranial arteries and scalp and facial capillaries all usually dilate, while the lumen of the internal carotid artery is narrowed.

There are many other factors which distinguish cluster headache from migraine, such as the predominantly male incidence, the pattern of recurrence and the brief duration of pain. These are listed in Table 13.2 which has been prepared from various publications (Anthony and

TABLE 13.2
Differences between migraine and 'cluster headache' (Lance and Anthony, 1971)

	Migraine	Cluster headache
Sex incidence (%)	female 75	male 85
Onset in childhood (%)	25	< 1
Unilateral pain (%)	65	100
Recurrence in bouts (%)	0	80
Frequency of attacks	$< 1-12$/month	1−8/day
Usual duration of pain	4−24 h	0·25−2 h
Associated features:		
nausea, vomiting (%)	85	45
blurring of vision (%)	common	8
lacrimation (%)	uncommon	85
blocked nostril (%)	uncommon	50
ptosis, miosis (%)	uncommon	25
hyperalgesia of face, scalp (%)	65	15
teichopsia, photopsia (%)	40	< 1
polyuria (%)	30	7
Past health:		
vomiting in childhood (%)	25	7
Family history:		
migraine (%)	50	20
Biochemical changes:		
fall in plasma serotonin (%)	80	0
rise in plasma histamine (%)	0	90
rise in CSF acetylcholine (%)	0	30

Lance, 1971; Ekbom, 1970; Lance and Anthony, 1966, 1971). The only factor in common between migraine and the syndrome under discussion is the dilatation of the extracranial arteries which has been observed at the height of the attack, and the relief of pain by drugs which constrict these vessels or prevent their dilatation. In every other respect, clinical and biochemical, the disorders differ, as outlined in Table 13.2. Apart from an occasional unexplained association with tic douloureux, there is no evidence that the condition has a neuralgic basis. It is therefore suggested that the misleading designation 'migrainous neuralgia' be replaced by the descriptive term 'cluster headache', until such time as the aetiology is fully understood. Exception can be taken to the use of 'cluster headache' on the grounds that about one-fifth of patients do not experience the typical periodicity of attacks implied by the name but the term is already accepted in medical literature and is more succinct and expressive than any alternative.

IS THIS SYNDROME OF HUMORAL ORIGIN?

Cluster headache is thus characterized by periodic vascular instability which is only rarely familial. If there is a primary disorder of humoral control of blood vessels, which chemical agents are involved? The syndrome is consistent with an excessive discharge of cholinergic nerve endings and it is of interest that Kunkle (1959) demonstrated an acetylcholine effect from cerebrospinal fluid specimens taken at the time of headache in 4 out of 14 patients with cluster headache which was not present in 7 patients with typical migraine. Plasma serotonin has been shown to fall during migraine headache, but does not alter significantly at the time of cluster headache (Anthony and Lance, 1971).

Since the reports by Horton and his colleagues, histamine has been considered as a possible mediator of cluster headache, although conventional anti-histaminic agents are not of value in treatment and the place of histamine desensitization is still controversial. Anthony and Lance (1971) reported that the mean blood level of histamine increased during cluster headache from 0.045 to 0.053 μg/ml ($P < 0.001$) but did not alter significantly in migraine headache. This finding differentiates cluster headache from migraine on biochemical as well as clinical grounds and renews interest in the possibility that histamine release plays some part in the symptomatology of cluster headache. It is tempting to think of the thickening of the wall of the internal carotid artery, which has been shown radiographically, as carotid 'hives' which causes intense pain by distension of the wall and compresses the pericarotid sympathetic plexus.

IS THIS SYNDROME OF NEURAL ORIGIN?

A neurogenic mechanism has been considered because of the sudden onset of pain, its brief duration and the association with lacrimation and blockage of the nostril.

Stimulation of the parasympathetic fibres travelling via the greater superficial petrosal nerve to the sphenopalatine ganglion evokes lacrimation and rhinorrhoea (Robinson, 1958) but transection of the greater superficial petrosal nerve has not prevented patients from having further attacks. White and Sweet (1955) stimulated the greater superficial petrosal nerve during craniotomy under local anaesthesia in 14 patients. Nine patients experienced pain localized to the ear, eye or adjacent parts of the head or face. After section of the nerve, pain could be elicited by stimulation of the central end only, indicating that the effect was mediated through afferent fibres and not indirectly by peripheral vasodilatation. The nerve was divided in 6 patients with cluster headache, but all experienced recurrence of pain at varying intervals postoperatively.

The stellate ganglion was blocked in 2 of our patients during a bout, producing a Horner's syndrome, but not provoking an attack. This suggests that a deficiency of sympathetic activity is not the primary factor. There have been no reports of any surgical operation preventing further bouts of cluster headache, although section of the trigeminal nerve will relieve the painful component of the attack arising from areas which it supplies.

In many instances pain involves the occipital area, neck or ear, areas supplied by the second and third cervical spinal segments. It is known that afferent fibres from the upper three cervical nerve roots make synaptic contact with neurones of the spinal nucleus of the trigeminal nerve in the upper cervical cord. It is therefore theoretically possible for a disturbance in this area to cause pain of both trigeminal and upper cervical distribution. A syndrome resembling cluster headache has been reported following whiplash injury to the neck in 8 patients (Hunter and Mayfield, 1949). Of our 60 patients 8 had experienced head injuries and the site of facial injury bore some relationship to the site of cluster headache in 4 patients. It is possible that injury to central or peripheral nervous pathways could cause vessels in the area of defective neurogenic control to become more susceptible to the action of humoral agents such as histamine. In view of male proneness to injury, this could explain why cluster headache is predominantly a male disease whereas migraine and tension headache are more common in women.

TREATMENT

The pain of cluster headache is so intense that patients understandably become apprehensive about the arrival of the next attack and may become depressed if their pain is not controlled. The effectiveness of treatment is difficult to assess because of possible variations in the length of each bout. Histamine desensitization was advocated before the natural history of the disorder was fully understood, so that a spontaneous remission was interpreted as a success for the treatment. The author has encountered patients who claimed that previous bouts had been stopped by histamine desensitization but who failed to gain relief when the same regimen was undertaken at the beginning of the next bout. With the recent demonstration of histamine release at the time of cluster headache, the value of antihistaminic agents must be reassessed. Failure of these agents in the past may have been related to their inability to counteract the action of tissue-bound histamine. There have been recent reports of pizotifen (Sandomigran), a potent antihistamine and antiserotonin agent, preventing further attacks of pain when taken in the dose of two 0·5 mg tablets three times daily during a bout.

In the absence of further knowledge of the mechanism of cluster headache, the most useful treatment is to attack one of the manifestations which gives rise to pain, dilatation of the extracranial arteries. The agents used are the same as for migraine but must be given regularly once, twice or three times each day, depending upon the times of the day when an attack of pain would be expected. In milder cases, oral preparations containing ergotamine tartrate such as Gynergen or Cafergot may be given as two tablets night and morning, or a Cafergot suppository may be inserted on retiring to bed if the attacks are solely nocturnal. If this fails, ergotamine tartrate, 0·5 mg, can be given by intramuscular injection at night, or twice daily, or methysergide can be administered orally in a dose of 2 mg three times daily. In some patients with severe cluster headache I have increased the dose of methysergide gradually to 12 to 15 mg daily before relief has been obtained. Provided the patient does not experience any side-effects (discussed in Chapter 12) as the dose is being increased, a high dosage of methysergide may be continued for the duration of the bout without cause for concern. As the anticipated end of the bout approaches, treatment should be ceased for a day to assess whether it is necessary to continue or not. If a characteristic attack ensues, then treatment is continued for another week before another test day of abstinence from medication. I have found methysergide and injected ergotamine tartrate each to be effective in about 70 per cent of patients.

Sjaastad and Dale (1974) reported 2 patients with a variant of cluster headache who experienced up to 12 to 18 attacks in 24 hours which responded to indomethacin, 50–75 mg daily, unlike most patients with this condition.

Following earlier reports by Graham that prednisone was of benefit in cluster headache, Jammes (1975) undertook a double-blind trial and found that a single dose of prednisone, 30 mg, was sufficient to relieve pain in 17 of 19 patients. Fourteen patients then remained free of pain for 60 days. Those in whom pain recurred were given prednisone, 20 mg daily, with significant relief of symptoms compared with those taking placebo tablets. Kudrow (1976) compared the success rates of methysergide, 8 mg daily, and prednisone, 40 mg daily, (reducing gradually over 21 days). Of 77 patients with typical episodic cluster headache, better than 75 per cent improvement was obtained in 41 patients on methysergide and 59 on prednisone. Of 15 patients with chronic cluster headache only 3 improved with methysergide while 11 improved with prednisone therapy. Kudrow also treated cases of chronic cluster headache with lithium carbonate, 600 mg daily, in two divided doses for 7 days, increasing to 900 mg daily for an additional two weeks with marked improvement in 13 of the 15 patients. From these reports it appears as though prednisone is an effective treatment for most bouts of cluster headache and that lithium carbonate is worthy of trial in chronic cluster headache. Patients maintained on lithium should have regular estimation of blood levels to minimize the risk of side-effects, the usual therapeutic range being 1 to 1.4 mEq/l.

The histamine-2 blocking agent, cimetidine, is at present undergoing clinical trials to assess its efficacy in cluster headache.

In patients resistant to all forms of pharmacotherapy, thermocoagulation of the Gasserian ganglion on the affected side should be considered, simply as a means of abolishing the pain of this severe disorder.

REFERENCES

Anthony, M. and Lance, J.W. (1971). Histamine and serotonin in cluster headache. *Archs. Neurol.* **25**, 225

Balla, J. I. and Walton J.N. (1964). Periodic migrainous neuralgia. *Br. med. J.* **1**, 219

Bickerstaff, E.R. (1959). The periodic migrainous neuralgia of Wilfred Harris. *Lancet* **1**, 1069

226   Cluster Headache (Migrainous Neuralgia)

226   Cluster Headache (Migrainous Neuralgia)

Broch, A., Hørven, I., Nornes, H., Sjaastad, O. and Tønjum, A. (1970). Studies on cerebral and ocular circulation in a patient with cluster headache. *Headache* **10**, 1.

Curran, D.A., Hinterberger, H. and Lance, J.W. (1967). Methysergide. *Res. clin. Stud. Headache* **1**, 74

Ekbom, K. (1970). A clinical comparison of cluster headache and migraine. *Acta neurol. scand.* **46**, (Suppl. 41), 1

Ekbom, K. and Greitz, T. (1970). Carotid angiography in cluster headache. *Acta radiol. (Diagn.)* **10**, 177

Friedman, A.P. and Mikropoulos, H.E. (1958). Cluster headaches. *Neurology, Minneap.* **8**, 653

Graham, J.R. (1972). Cluster headache. *Headache* **11**, 175

Harris, W. (1936). Ciliary (migrainous) neuralgia and its treatment. *Br. med. J.* **1**, 457

Horton, B.J., MacLean, A.R. and Craig, W. McK. (1939). A new syndrome of vascular headache: results of treatment with histamine: preliminary report. *Proc. Staff Meet. Mayo Clin.* **14**, 257

Hørven, I., Nornes, H. and Sjaastad, O. (1972). Different corneal indentation pulse pattern in cluster headache and migraine. *Neurology* **22**, 92

Hunter, C.R. and Mayfield, F.H. (1949). Role of the upper cervical roots in the production of pain in the head *Am. J. Surg.* **78**, 743

Jammes, J.L. (1975). The treatment of cluster headaches with prednisone. *Dis. nerv. Syst.* **36**, 375

Kudrow, L. (1976). Comparative results of prednisone, methysergide and lithium therapy in cluster headache. *Abstracts, International symposium,* Sept. 16–17, p. 15. London: Migraine Trust

Kunkle, E.C. (1959). Acetylcholine in the mechanism of headaches of the migraine type. *Archs Neurol. Psychiat., Chicago* **84**, 135

Kunkle, E.C. and Anderson, W.B. (1961). Significance of minor eye signs in headache of migraine type. *Archs Ophthal., Chicago* **65**, 504

Kunkle, E.C., Pfeiffer, J.B., Wilhoit, W.M. and Lamrick, L.W. (1954). Recurrent brief headaches in 'cluster' pattern. *N. Carol. med. J.* **15**, 510

Lance, J.W. and Anthony, M. (1966). Some clinical aspects of migraine. *Archs Neurol.* **15**, 356

Lance, J.W. and Anthony, M. (1971). Migrainous neuralgia or cluster headache? *J. Neurol. Sci.* **13**, 401

Nieman, E.A. and Hurwitz, L.J. (1961). Ocular sympathetic palsy in periodic migrainous neuralgia. *J. Neurol. Neurosurg. Psychiat.* **24**, 369

Robinson, B.W. (1958). Histaminic cephalgia. *Medicine, Baltimore* **37**, 161

Romberg, M.H. (1840). *A Manual of Nervous Diseases of Man.* Transl. E. H. Sieveking. London: Sydenham Society

Sjaastad, O. and Dale, I. (1974). Evidence of a new (?) treatable headache entity. *Headache* **14**, 105

Sluder, G. (1910). The syndrome of sphenopalatine-ganglion neurosis. *Am. J. med. Sci.* **140**, 868

Sutherland, J.M. and Eadie, M.J. (1972). Cluster headache. In *Res. clin. Stud. Headache,* **3**, 92

Symonds, C.P. (1956). A particular variety of headache. *Brain* **79**, 217

Vail, H.H. (1932). Vidian neuralgia. *Ann. Otol. Rhinol. Lar.* **41**, 837

White, J. and Sweet, W. (1955). *Pain. Its Mechanism and Neurosurgical Control.* Springfield: Thomas

Wood, E.H. and Friedman, A.P. (1976). Thermography in cluster headache. *Res. clin. Stud. Headache.* **4**, 107

Fourteen
Post-Traumatic Headache

The incidence of post-traumatic headache varies in different series from 33 to 80 per cent. The problem which exercises the neurologist is to asssign the correct proportion of organic and psychological factors in each particular instance. Brenner *et al.* (1944) found that post-traumatic headache lasting more than 2 months was uncommon in those patients who were only dazed and were not disorientated after the injury, and those without post-traumatic amnesia. It was significantly higher in those with laceration of the scalp and in those of a nervous disposition before the accident, with symptoms of anxiety after the accident or with occupational difficulties or pending litigation. There was no correlation with the duration of coma, disorientation or post-traumatic amnesia when these were present, or with EEG abnormalities during the first week, skull fracture or the finding of blood in the CSF. These authors quote earlier work by Friedman and Brenner which showed that patients with localized post-traumatic headache were very sensitive to intravenous histamine which reproduced the characteristic headache. These findings suggest that some post-traumatic headache is of intracranial origin (worsened by histamine), some is of extracranial origin (following laceration of the scalp), and some is of psychosomatic origin (worsened by anxiety and concern about litigation).

Simons and Wolff (1946) found that the intravenous injection of 0·1 to 0·2 mg histamine in 16 patients with post-traumatic headache gave rise to a deep ache, sometimes throbbing, which was most intensive in the occipital and frontal regions. The sensitivity of the patients to histamine was no greater than that of normal subjects but in 3 cases the headache was most intense at the site of head injury. They divided post-traumatic headache into three groups. The first was a dull

227

pressure sensation, associated with nervous tension and depression, in which EMG recordings from the scalp muscles correlated with the severity of headache. The injection of local anaesthetic into areas of deep tenderness reduced or abolished the headache. They concluded that this form resulted from sustained contraction of skeletal muscle. The second variety of headache was a local pain and tenderness in an area of scarring which was superimposed on a generalized dull headache of the first type. The third variety was a unilateral throbbing headache with nausea, accompanied by dilatation of arteries and veins and relieved by ergotamine. This is referred to below as extracranial vascular headache or post-traumatic migraine. This study thus emphasized the importance of extracranial structures in producing the headache, whether or not there was an underlying neurosis. It emphasized that legal procedures should be settled promptly in case the symptoms, including headache, are indefinitely prolonged.

The settlement of the legal aspects of the matter does not always lead to disappearance of symptoms and return to work. Balla and Moraitis (1970) followed up 82 patients, 41 of whom suffered from headache, after industrial or traffic accidents. They found that 21 patients had not returned to work 2 years after financial settlement. Those who did return to work usually did so within a year.

Ellard (1970) has summarized the psychological reactions he has encountered in patients with a compensable injury as follows:

Attitudinal pathosis

A patient who does not seek to be healed but to be justified. He is not incapacitated by symptoms but has a grievance and believes that he cannot work because he has been dealt with unjustly.

Schizophrenic reaction

This is commonly paranoid with feelings of persecution by doctors, solicitors and even the law courts. Less commonly, a neurotic illness develops extraordinary features, such as the man who had a bump on the head and thereafter wore glasses with one red lens and one green lens and could walk only with the aid of a stick adorned by a wheel at one end and a bicycle bell at the other. Ellard comments that patients who habitually wear pyjama trousers under their ordinary trousers seem to pursue a particularly malignant course.

Bizarre hypochondriasis

A group of patients who before injury were fitness fanatics, narcissistic and preoccupied with health foods and sporting activities. They commonly describe their headache in an exaggerated manner and are often diagnosed as hysterical.

Traumatic neurosis

Here the accident may have symbolic significance, perhaps of a sexual nature, but more commonly the patient's anxiety is conditioned by the accident, like the woman who could only tolerate being driven in a car if she huddled under a rug in the rear compartment drinking brandy. Such patients may respond to behaviour therapy.

Depression

Many patients who become depressed are of compulsive personality in whom work has become an important defence mechanism. Typical depressive symptoms follow deprivation of their normal working pattern.

Compensation neurosis

Depressive symptoms are usually overshadowed by those of anxiety. The patient often becomes aggressive at work as well as at home. Hysterical manifestations may become superimposed. The total amount of disability is usually greater than the sum of its parts.

Malingering

The paradox of the man who remains sick because of the hope of financial reward.

Ellard stresses the need to assess each patient in the light of his racial, cultural and educational background as well as his premorbid personality. The patient with an excessive psychological reaction to injury looks well in spite of his description of suffering. There is a lack of motivation to get well and his attitude to treatment is unusual and may be resentful.

In the present state of knowledge, headache following injury cannot be classified with certainty in any one group. It is probable that there are at least five distinct types of post-traumatic headache, with overlap between the groups.

(1) Intracranial vascular headache

It is generally accepted that concussion is followed by dilatation of intracranial vessels, giving rise to a pulsating headache which is made worse by head movement, jolting, coughing, sneezing and straining. In fact this applies to a minority of patients. Tubbs and Potter (1970) found that only 83 of 200 patients admitted to hospital had a headache in the day or so after head injury. Headache was complained of spontaneously by 22 patients (11 per cent), of whom 3 required an analgesic. The remainder admitted to headache only on questioning. Sensitivity to jolting, coughing or straining may persist in some patients without any obvious neurological signs being present. It may be associated with other symptoms of organic origin, such as giddiness on looking upwards or on lying down with the head to one side or the other (benign positional vertigo). The same type of headache may develop, or intensify, in the case of subdural haematoma arising as a result of head injury.

(2) Extracranial vascular headache

It is not uncommon for patients who have experienced local damage to the scalp overlying a main extracranial vessel to become subject to periodic headache in the distribution of that vessel. Such headaches have been called post-traumatic migraine, since they recur with the periodicity of migraine and may be associated with nausea and photophobia. Jabbing pains may also rise from any scalp nerve damaged by the blow, or subsequent development of scar tissue. Ligation and section of the affected nerve and vessel may be helpful in abolishing this syndrome. Apart from surgical measures, the management is the same as for migraine.

(3) Post-traumatic dysautonomic cephalalgia

Vijayan and Dreyfus (1975) described 5 patients with a distinctive syndrome which followed injury to the anterior triangle of the neck, presumably involving the carotid artery sheath. All patients complained of pain and tenderness in this area for some weeks after the injury. Some weeks or months after the injury the patients began to suffer from severe unilateral episodic headaches on the side previously injured. The headaches were frontotemporal in site associated with severe sweating over the same side of the face, dilatation of the pupil on that side, blurring of vision and photophobia in the ipsilateral eye, and nausea. The headaches recurred several times each month and lasted 8 hours to 3 days. After the headache subsided 3 patients were said to have ptosis and miosis on the affected side. The attacks were attributed to a paroxysmal excess of sympathetic activity followed by a period of diminished activity, as a result of trauma to the pericarotid sympathetic plexus. Partial sympathetic denervation was confirmed by the fact that the pupil on the affected side dilated in response to a 1:1 000 solution of adrenaline. The headaches did not improve with ergotamine but responded promptly to propranolol, 40 mg daily.

(4) Pain in the neck and occipital region from injury to the upper cervical spine

The part played by whiplash injury of the cervical spine is difficult to assess in the absence of definite radiological changes. Dr J.I. Balla of Melbourne (unpublished data) has analysed the symptoms attributed to whiplash injury in 300 patients, two-thirds of whom were female, examined six months or more after the accident which was considered to be responsible. Daily aching in the neck was a complaint of 219 patients and 58 had aching in the arms. Headache recurred daily in 176 patients (59 per cent), every week or so in 42 patients (14 per cent) and occasionally or not at all in 82 patients (27 per cent). The daily headaches were described as a generalized ache, worse toward the back of the head. Those patients with occasional or weekly headaches resembled those with common migraine. More work is required to establish which components of the whiplash syndrome are caused by damage to cervical discs, ligaments or soft tissues, and which are caused by excessive muscle contraction associated with anxiety and depression.

Referral of pain from the upper cervical roots to the head has been discussed in Chapter 1 and in the section on the neck in Chapter 6. After cervical disc injury, the neck may be held in a slightly tilted or rigidly fixed position. Points of referred tenderness are often found, not only in the suboccipital and cervical regions but over the upper part of the medial edge of the scapula, the deltoid muscle and around the elbow on the affected side (Raney and Raney, 1948). Some patients respond to the application of heat and cervical traction, some to manipulation of the neck and some to the injection of a local anaesthetic agent and hydrocortisone into tender areas of the suboccipital region of the neck. Relaxation training is a useful adjunct to other forms of treatment because muscle contraction or 'spasm' is commonly present. Psychological management and the use of antidepressants may be equally important.

Paroxysmal unilateral headaches resembling cluster headache were reported by Hunter and Mayfield (1949) to follow trauma in 8 patients. The headaches resembled cluster headaches in that they came on at night, and were accompanied by lacrimation, blockage of the nostril, flushing and abnormal sweating on the side of the headache. Pupillary changes were not mentioned. The pain was said to cease abruptly when the second cervical root was anaesthetized and to disappear completely when this root was sectioned. Follow-up was brief and the suspicion remains that the authors were simply observing the usual intermittent pattern of cluster headaches.

(5) Muscle-contraction ('tension') headache

It has been amply pointed out in the medical literature that multiple symptoms may follow minor head injuries where compensation or litigation is involved and that self-employed or professional men return to work more rapidly than employees after head injury, and that sporting injuries are not usually followed by disability. Any tendency to anxiety or depression appears to be accentuated by head injury, and the personality of the patient before the accident plays a large part in the way that he reacts to injury. Some post-traumatic headaches have all the qualities of tension headache and respond, at least in part, to the use of tranquillizing and antidepressant drugs. The tendency to this form of headache is often engendered by that natural worry which attaches to the possibility of brain damage and is reinforced by some legal advisors who instruct their clients not to resume work or normal activities until the case is settled. The concept of accident neurosis has been discussed in detail in two lectures by Miller (1961).

The early management of head injury may be important in reducing the disability which so often follows. Relander and his colleagues (1972) compared the result of an active treatment programme with the routine treatment of comparable patients in the same hospital. The active treatment group were visited daily and the nature of the injury was explained to them. They were encouraged to get out of bed and start physiotherapy. When they attended the follow-up clinic, they were seen by the same doctors who had looked after them in hospital. The active treatment group returned to work in an average of 18 days compared with 32 days for other patients.

The great difficulty in handling patients with post-traumatic headache is to differentiate the organic from the psychogenic components. It seems undeniable that some post-traumatic headache is of organic origin, in the sense that the control of cranial vessels has become more unstable, and cranial arteries have become more susceptible to painful dilatation since injury (Taylor, 1967). It requires an unbiased approach on the part of the physician and a careful assessment of each patient's personality and his headache pattern to ensure that justice is done to his legal claim and that treatment is appropriate to his variety of headache.

REFERENCES

Balla, J.I. and Moraitis, S. (1970). Knights in armour. A follow-up study of injuries after legal settlement. *Med. J. Aust.* **2**, 355

Brenner, C., Friedman, A.P., Merritt, H.H. and Denny-Brown, D.E. (1944). Post-traumatic headache. *J. Neurosurg.* **6**, 379

Ellard, J. (1970). Psychological reactions to compensable injury. *Med. J. Aust.* **2**, 349

Hunter, C.R. and Mayfield, F.H. (1949). Role of the upper cervical roots in the production of pain in the head. *Am. J. Surg.* **78**, 743

Miller, H. (1961). Accident neurosis. *Br. med. J.* **1**, 919, 992

Raney, A.A. and Raney, R.B. (1948). Headache: a common symptom of cervical disk lesions. *Archs. Neurol. Psychiat. Chicago.* **59**, 603

Relander, M., Troupp, H., and Björkesten, G. af. (1972). Controlled trial of treatment for cervical concussion. *Br. med. J.* **2**, 777

Simons, D.J. and Wolff, H.G. (1946). Studies on headache: mechanisms of chronic post-traumatic headache. *Psychosom. Med.* **8**, 227

Taylor, A.R. (1967). Post-concussional sequelae. *Br. med. J.* **2**, 67

Tubbs, O.N. and Potter, J.M. (1970). Early post-concussional headache. *Lancet* **2**, 128

Vijayan, N. and Dreyfus, P.M. (1975). Post-traumatic dysautonomic cephalalgia, clinical observations and treatment. *Archs Neurol.* **32**, 649

Fifteen

The Investigation and Management of Headache Problems

When you're lying awake with a dismal headache,
and repose is taboo'd by anxiety,
I conceive you may use any language you choose
To indulge in, without impropriety.

Iolanthe, *W. S. Gilbert*

A headache, at best, is an unpleasant thing. It is more unpleasant because it attacks the seat of reason, and there are few patients with headache who are not troubled by thoughts of cerebral tumour or intracranial disaster. For the doctor to be able to reassure his patient, he must have a clear idea of the diagnosis, based on clinical judgment and supported when necessary by special investigations.

The initial problem in management is the decision as to whether any special investigation is warranted. In the majority of patients, a careful history will establish the pattern so clearly that any special tests are superfluous. When there is diagnostic difficulty or when the history suggests a serious disorder, investigation becomes obligatory, and judgment is required to determine the sequence of tests which is safest for the patient and most likely to produce a definitive answer.

The clinical approach will depend upon the duration of headache and its mode of presentation.

234

The acute severe headache

When a headache suddenly develops in a patient for the first time, the presence or absence of fever and neck rigidity is of great importance. Patients with acute headache, photophobia, elevation of body temperature and neck stiffness obviously have an intracranial disturbance, and the question of lumbar puncture arises. If there are other signs of one of the infectious fevers then lumbar puncture can be deferred. The CSF commonly shows a lymphocytic pleocytosis if headache is present at the height of a viral invasion but this knowledge does not assist in management. When a confident diagnosis of a specific infection cannot be made after examination of the patient, lumbar puncture may be necessary to distinguish between meningitis, encephalitis and subarachnoid haemorrhage. The normal CSF should not contain more than 5 lymphocytes/mm^3 and should never contain polymorphonuclear cells. A high polymorph count is almost always caused by bacterial meningitis and a purely lymphocytic reaction indicates a viral meningoencephalitis, but mixed cellular reactions may be found in both viral and bacterial infections, particularly in tuberculous meningitis. The glucose content of CSF assumes particular significance in these doubtful cases. The CSF level of glucose depends upon the blood level but, providing that the patient is not hypoglycaemic and that the fluid has not been allowed to stand for some hours before examination, a CSF glucose of 30 mg/100 ml (2 mmol/l) or less suggests a bacterial or cryptococcal meningitis, or the rare meningitis carcinomatosa.

Apart from the diagnosis of infectious disease, lumbar puncture may be required to confirm this diagnosis of subarachnoid haemorrhage. If the diagnosis of subarachnoid haemorrhage is self-evident and the patient is conscious, it is often better to proceed immediately to cerebral angiography in a centre which is suitably equipped, since lumbar puncture gives no additional information and may precipitate further bleeding.

After head injury, there may be difficulty in distinguishing postconcussional vascular headache from that of an expanding intracranial haematoma. A unilateral headache and insidious drowsiness are always signals to be on the alert. Dilatation of one pupil or a minimal hemiparesis are late signs which should prompt immediate carotid angiography and neurosurgical intervention. Neck stiffness arising in this context is a particular source of concern as it suggests mid-brain compression from 'coning' of one temporal lobe through the tentorial opening. When radiography of the skull demonstrates a fracture of the lateral aspect, the possibility of an extradural haematoma from a torn middle meningeal artery should be borne in mind, and justifies close observation of the patient. A computerized axial tomogram (CT scan) is particularly helpful in following the course of patients with a post-traumatic headache of doubtful origin.

Acute headaches without neck stiffness may also be of intracranial origin. Blood pressure may suddenly increase in acute nephritis, toxaemia of pregnancy, malignant hypertension, and the crises caused by phaeochromocytoma or by a patient on mono-amine oxidase inhibitors taking sympathomimetic drugs or tyramine-containing foods. The latter syndrome will probably become more common with the increasing use of MAO inhibitors for depression. The finding of hypertension on examination does not of course mean that the patient does not have an intracranial lesion as the source of headache. The blood pressure is usually secondarily elevated in patients with subarachnoid and intracerebral haemorrhage.

Acute headaches of extracranial origin (sinusitis, retrobulbar neuritis, acute angle-closure glaucoma and abscesses around the roots of the upper teeth) can usually be diagnosed clinically.

Acute recurrent episodes of headaches

Some of the entities mentioned above (sinusitis, pressor reaction of phaeochromocytoma) may recur periodically. Repeated episodes of meningitis suggest either defective immunological mechanisms or, more commonly, that the nasopharynx communicates with the subarachnoid space through a fracture in the floor of the anterior fossa. This leads to CSF rhinorrhoea, with clear fluid dripping from the nostril when the head is bent forwards. CSF, unlike nasal secretions, contains glucose so that a Clinistix dipped into the nostril can rapidly confirm that the fluid is of intracranial origin. The fistula can be repaired surgically with a fascial graft.

Repetition of a subarachnoid haemorrhage from intracranial aneurysm carries a mortality in the vicinity of 50 per cent, like that of the original episode. Cerebral, cerebellar or spinal angiomas on the other hand may bleed 'little and often' throughout life, with little or no residual deficit. Angiomas can be dealt with surgically if their arterial supply is accessible, but in other cases any surgical procedure could cause more havoc than the natural history of the disease, so that the patient is advised to ride out each storm as it comes.

Attacks of cerebrovascular insufficiency are clearly demarcated by symptoms and signs of the territory which is rendered ischaemic. The classic story of internal carotid insufficiency, usually seen only in part, is that of blurring of vision in one eye (resulting from retinal ischaemia) accompanied by fleeting paraesthesiae or paresis of the opposite side. If the dominant hemisphere (the left in right-handed subjects; either or both in left-handed patients) is involved, dysphasia is an additional symptom. Transient ischaemic attacks may be accompanied by headache on the side supplied by the defective carotid artery. Insufficiency of the vertebrobasilar artery is characterized by momentary vertigo, dysarthria and ataxia, or by a mélange of brainstem symptoms and signs, including diplopia, tinnitus, deafness, paraesthesiae over the face and body and hemiparesis or quadriparesis. Because the posterior cerebral arteries, which supply the occipital cortex, arise from the basilar artery, the patient may experience a temporary homonymous hemianopia, visual hallucinations like those of migraine, or a complete bilateral suppression of vision. Since the medial part of the temporal lobe, which is the entry portal of the brain for memory, is also within the distribution of the posterior cerebral artery, amnesia may be a feature of vertebrobasilar attacks. The occipital headache, which may be present for the duration of the attack, is insignificant compared with the dramatic nature of the focal neurological symptoms.

The investigation of cerebral vascular insufficiency is beyond the scope of this book, but it is worth emphasizing that the history and examination may indicate the underlying cause of the attacks. Paroxysmal cardiac dysrhythmias may produce the attacks through hypotension, sudden neck movements may obliterate the lumen of the vertebral artery in the neck of spondylitic patients, and arm movements may induce a shunting of blood from the vertebral artery into the subclavian artery if its intraluminal pressure is lowered because of stenosis in the first part of the vessel. Inequality of the radial pulses and a bruit over the clavicles or in the neck may indicate the site of stenoses in major vessels.

Intermittent hydrocephalus is a rare cause of recurrent headache, but should be considered if the history is relatively short, if the headaches are severe, if they are precipitated by a quick forward movement of the head, or are associated with obscuration of vision, impairment of consciousness, myoclonic jerks or weakness of the legs. The final diagnosis will depend upon CT scanning and other neurological investigations.

The pattern of pain or headache in tic douloureux, cluster headache and migraine has been considered at some length earlier in this book and is usually sufficiently distinctive for a diagnosis to be made (*Figure 15.1*). Where doubt exists, other conditions may be excluded by investigations, but a positive diagnosis depends upon the clinical story. The diagnosis of migraine is supported by the finding of a low plasma level of serotonin at the time of a headache. This cannot be used as a routine test for migraine because most laboratories do not estimate serotonin often enough for accurate results to be obtained, and because plasma serotonin varies so much between individuals that a baseline level has to be established for that particular patient before the level in the headache samples can be interpreted.

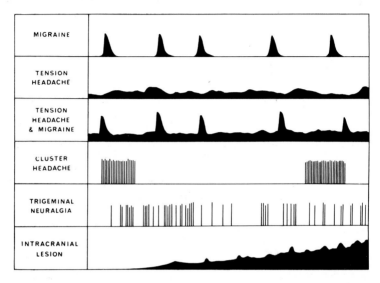

Figure 15.1. Temporal patterns of headache discussed in Chapter 4. This scheme does not bring out the difference in duration between the pain of trigeminal neuralgia (repeated jabs lasting a fraction of a second) and that of cluster headache (each lasting 20 to 120 minutes)

Migraine may be accompanied by any of the symptoms which were mentioned in the description of cerebral vascular insufficiency. Indeed, these features of migraine may be regarded as a prolonged ischaemia of internal carotid or vertebrobasilar territory. The duration of focal neurological symptoms in migraine commonly varies from 10 to 30 minutes, but there are instances in which they may be prolonged for hours or days, or keep recurring intermittently for weeks, as 'status migrainosus vasospasticus'. One patient aged 26 years has experienced several episodes of recurring bilateral scintillating scotomas and left homonymous hemianopia lasting up to 2 weeks, associated with numbness, weakness and continuous epileptic jerking of the left side of the body on one occasion, and dysarthria, inco-ordination of the right hand, ataxia and stupor on another. Residual deficits have taken some months to resolve. The associated headache has been unilateral, commonly left-sided. It is only after years of observation and repeated investigations that this syndrome can confidently be regarded as a variant of migraine.

The fact that different areas of brain or brainstem have been involved on different occasions, that the headache has varied from right to left, and that the headache has at times been on the side inappropriate for the initiation of the focal symptoms, all favour the diagnosis of migraine, and may be helpful in assessing symptoms which could be caused either by migrainous vasospasm or by a fixed intracranial lesion.

Headache of subacute onset

This group is of interest to the doctor and of potential danger to the patient. Someone who has never experienced more than 'ordinary headaches', which most of us get at times, starts to complain of a different sort of headache which may affect one or both sides and becomes progressively more severe. If the patient has been complaining of earache, or of nasal obstruction with pain over the forehead or maxillae before the onset of headache, thoughts turn to the intracranial complications of otitis media and sinusitis.

If the patient has signs of raised intracranial pressure, the EEG is very useful in deciding whether a focal lesion such as a cerebral abscess is present (*see Figure 6.4*). If a CT scanner is not available, a carotid angiogram will determine whether the lateral ventricles are large or small. If the lateral ventricles are not enlarged and there is no displacement of vessels, it is safe to introduce air through a lumbar puncture needle to delineate the ventricular system by pneumo-encephalography. If the ventricles are large there is probably an obstructive hydrocephalus and it is safer for a neurosurgeon to drain the lateral ventricles and later find the site of obstruction by injecting air or a radio-opaque substance into the ventricular system.

The rare case of Addison's disease or hypocalcaemia presenting with increased intracranial pressure must be remembered and excluded.

Electroencephalography, radionuclide and CT scanning are also of great assistance when tumour or subdural haematoma is suspected. The EEG is abnormal in the majority of patients with these conditions and can indicate the probable side and position of the lesion in most cases so that carotid arteriography can be done on the appropriate side. The radionuclide or CT scan may outline precisely the site of tumour or haematoma.

In patients over the age of 55 years the blood picture and erythrocyte sedimentation rate should always be examined to pick up the odd patient with temporal arteritis.

Chronic headache

In the patient who has suffered from headaches for a year or more, the prospect of a tumour or other serious intracranial disorder being the cause is more remote, but one cannot be completely sure unless the duration of the patient's headaches is more than 5 years. If the patient's headaches have been consistent in character for 5 years or more one may feel fairly confident that they are not caused by intracranial tumour, although the occasional patient may be found to have a tumour which is quite unrelated to the headache with which he presented. The author recalls a patient with a pituitary tumour who complained of a typical tension headache, which responded well to treatment in spite of its duration of 20 years. The author missed the significance of her appearance and did not investigate further. Some time later she presented with bilateral carpal-tunnel syndrome, induced by acromegaly, when the diagnosis of pituitary tumour was finally made. The author remains convinced that her headache was not caused by her tumour.

Of the 1152 patients who attended a clinic for chronic headache, only 1 was found to have a cerebral tumour. The diagnosis was made by finding intracranial calcification on radiography of the skull, which was done to reassure the patient, whose symptoms were those of tension headache.

As a general rule, any headache which has been present for more than 5 years is a muscle-contraction headache or migraine.

THE INVESTIGATION OF HEADACHE

Only a small percentage of patients with headache requires any investigation other than a careful history and examination.

Blood count and erthyrocyte sedimentation rate (ESR)

These are routine tests for patients admitted to hospital and should be done in general practice when there have been symptoms of systemic disorder, or signs of infection or meningeal reaction associated with headache, or when dealing with a patient above the age of 55 years in whom the possibility of temporal arteritis must be ruled out. Polycy- thaemia may be the result of arteriovenous shunting as in cerebral angioma, haemangioblastoma of the cerebellum and Paget's disease. Leukaemia may present with intracranial deposits. Anaemia may indicate neoplasia or other systemic disease, and may accentuate any tendency to headache. A high ESR often directs attention to some locus of infection, hidden malignancy or an unusual condition such as myelomatosis, one of the collagen diseases or subacute bacterial endo- carditis, which may all produce intracranial manifestations.

Lumbar puncture

Some recent medical graduates assume that a lumbar puncture must be done in any patient complaining of neurological symptoms, and await each new admission with needle poised. If there were such a concept as a 'routine neurological work-up', which fortunately there is not, lumbar puncture would not usually form part of it. There are specific indica- tions for lumbar puncture, and suspected intracranial tumour is not one of them. If there is genuine suspicion of cerebral tumour, radionuclide and CT scan or contrast radiographic studies will be necessary to attempt to localize or exclude it. A sample of CSF can be taken at the beginning of pneumo-encephalography although really it helps little to know whether fluid constituents, such as protein, vary slightly from normal. Lumbar puncture is used in the investigation of headache to confirm the presence of subarachnoid haemorrhage, to investigate infectious processes of the nervous system, including syphilis, or to measure intracranial pressure in benign intracranial hypertension.

There is a modern tendency to decry the hazards of lumbar puncture in the presence of papilloedema, but it is potentially dangerous unless a CT scan or carotid angiography has shown that there is no internal hydrocephalus or displacement of midline structures. Should lumbar puncture have to be done without this safeguard in a patient with raised intracranial pressure, in, for example, a patient with bilateral papilloe- dema who is suspected of having bacterial meningitis, it is a worthwhile precaution to have a 20-ml syringe filled with normal saline solution which can be injected intrathecally should any untoward symptoms follow the withdrawal of CSF.

A small point concerning the technique of lumbar puncture which the author has found useful, is to infiltrate the skin with local anaesthetic 1–2 cm laterally to the midline at the selected interver- tebral disc space and to angulate the lumbar puncture needle towards the midline as it is inserted from this point. The suggested track passes through soft tissues until the needle touches the spine. A gentle tapping movement of the needle will indicate to the examiner whether the needle is in contact with bone or with the elastic interlaminar ligament. If the latter, the needle can be inserted through the ligament with confidence that CSF will emerge when the stilette is removed. The advantages of this lateral approach are that it is usually painless and permits tactile sensibility of the position of the needle point. These advantages are lost with the firm pressure required to penetrate the interspinous ligament in the midline approach, making it difficult to know when the lumbar sac is entered.

Electroencephalography

The EEG can give only a limited range of answers to any clinical question, but is a most useful investigation because it is painless, harmless and relatively inexpensive. It may give a complete answer in some conditions such as intracranial abscess, which gives rise to an angry focus of slow waves (*see Figure 6.4*). It may also give an accurate localization in cerebral tumour, but regrettably the most striking EEG foci are produced by the most rapidly growing and malignant tumours, and a benign tumour of long-standing, such as a meningioma, may not alter the tracing at all. Lateralizing abnormalities may indicate a lesion such as subdural haematoma which interferes with the recording of the normal electrical activity of the brain and induces slow rhythms from the surrounding area of the brain which is compressed. The changes produced by diffuse disorders, such as meningitis, encephalitis, or metabolic disturbances are of little diagnostic value. It is generally agreed that the proportion of abnormal tracings found in migraine is higher than in the general population, but the changes are non-specific (Goldensohn, 1976) and are probably secondary to repeated attacks of cerebral ischaemia (Slatter, 1968). The EEG is most useful in the patient whose headaches do not fit any particular pattern, as a partial reassurance against the presence of a space-occupying lesion; or in the patient who is suspected of harbouring such a lesion but has no lateralizing symptoms or signs, as a preliminary to special radiographic investigations. The EEG may give a clear indication of the side of the lesion, and thus guide the clinician to the side to be examined by carotid angiography. It may also be of indirect benefit in patients with tension headache by disclosing muscle artefact which persists over the site of muscle contraction (*Figure 15.2*).

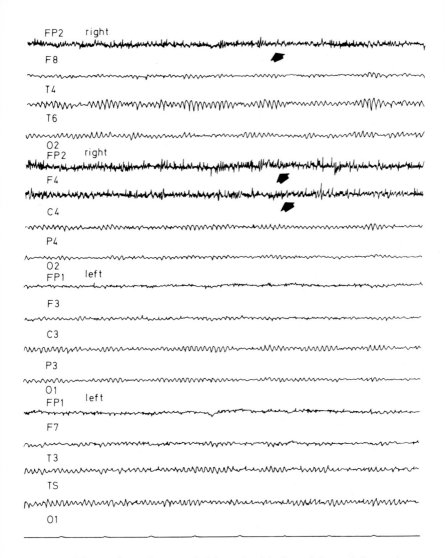

Figure 15.2. Muscle artefact recorded from the right frontal electrode in a patient with persistent headache over the right frontotemporal region

Plain radiography

The patient whose headache is sufficiently troublesome to warrant radiography of the skull should always have a film of the chest taken at the same time. There are many ways in which diseases of the heart and lungs may affect the brain. Pulmonary tuberculosis may be associated with tuberculous meningitis, bronchiectasis with cerebral abscess and carcinoma of the lung with cerebral metastases.

Radiography of the skull is an essential stage in the diagnosis of headaches which do not fit into a recognizable benign pattern. The pituitary fossa is first inspected in the lateral films and then the vault is surveyed systematically, looking for fractures, areas of radiolucency or sclerosis. The angle which the horizontal plane of the axis makes with the hard palate is examined to ensure that there is no platybasia (basilar impression), which has been illustrated in *Figure 8.8*.

Calcification is noted in the normal sites: pineal gland and habenular trigone, choroid plexuses and petroclinoid ligaments. Abnormal calcification is sought, particularly above the pituitary fossa, the common site for a craniopharyngioma. The sinuses and mastoid air cells are inspected. The shadow of the pharyngeal tissue is examined if the question of nasopharyngeal carcinoma has arisen.

In the anteroposterior projections, the position of the pineal gland, if calcified, is checked and any displacement from the midline noted. Any abnormal calcification is localized. The sphenoid wings and the posterior clinoid processes are examined. The sinuses are again examined. In the Towne's view, the internal auditory meatus can be seen clearly on each side. If the patient has a nerve deafness then Stenver's views or tomography of the internal auditory meatus are essential. The basal view of the skull should be searched for fractures, erosions, enlargement of the jugular foramen, foramen ovale or foramen spinosum. The latter may enlarge on the same side as a vascular meningioma because it is traversed by the middle meningeal artery.

Opinions differ about the significance of certain findings. Hyperostosis frontalis interna is regarded by some European authors as an inflammatory condition producing headache. It is a common variation of normal from middle-age onwards, particularly in female patients, and the author is unaware of any controlled observations linking it with headache. 'Thumbing', a beaten-copper appearance of the cranial vault, may be a normal variation, although it alerts the observer to the possibility of long-standing raised intracranial pressure (*see Figure 8.8*). The sutures should be observed carefully in the young child as they separate when intracranial pressure is increased.

In most patients with headache, the appearance of the skull radiograph will be normal but a surprise turns up often enough to make the procedure worthwhile. The most useful facet of skull radiography is often the position of the pineal gland. It must be remembered, however, that midline structures are not always displaced by cerebral tumour, and that a pineal gland remains central with bilateral symmetrical subdural haematomas.

Echo-encephalography

The echo-encephalograph is a device which is useful in those subjects who are unfortunate enough to have a pineal gland which is uncalcified. The technique is being developed so as to pick up information other than the midline 'echo', such as the position and size of the ventricles and the localization of intracerebral tumours, but at the time of writing other methods give this information more precisely. Echo-encephalography is only of value if the recordist is expert in its use.

Radionuclide brain studies (isotope scanning, brain scintigraphy)

This form of scanning requires the intravenous injection of a radioactive isotope, usually $^{99}Tc^m$ pertechnetate. The passage of isotope through the carotid arteries and their middle cerebral and anterior cerebral branches is recorded by a gamma camera as a 'dynamic scan' (cerebral nuclide angiogram, CRAG). Flow can be measured precisely by means of a computer. Dynamic scanning will demonstrate impairment of blood flow in the carotid circulation and is therefore a useful and safe preliminary investigation in patients with presumed cerebral vascular disease.

After the dynamic phase, a static scan demonstrates any area of abnormal isotope accumulation. This stage may be delayed for 2 to 3 hours if the uptake into the suspected lesion is slow, for example metastases and chronic subdural haematoma. Abnormality is demonstrated when there is disruption of the blood–brain barrier. The technique detects 80 to 85 per cent of supratentorial neoplasms (*Figure 15.3a*) and 70 to 75 per cent of infratentorial neoplasms. It will pick up virtually all cerebral abscesses, most subdural haematomas of more than 3 weeks duration (*Figure 15.3b*) and most angiomas. The static scan becomes positive several days after cerebral infarction and remains abnormal for about 6 weeks. Isotope scans are of no value in atrophic lesions.

Any form of isotope study is best avoided during pregnancy.

TABLE 15.1
Table for differential diagnosis of headache

	Site	Photophobia	Neck stiffness	Worse on jolting	Drowsiness	Focal symptoms and signs	EEG	Skull radiograph	CSF	Arteriogram or CT scan
ACUTE SINGLE EPISODES (minutes or hours)										
Subarachnoid haem.	1	+	+	+	+	cer. or b.s.	occ. focal	–	blood-stained	aneurysm angioma
Encephalitis	1	+	+	+	+	cer. or b.s.	nonspec.	–	mainly lympho-cytic.	–
Meningitis	1	+	+	+	+	–	nonspec.	–	mainly p.m.n.	–
Post-concussion	1	+	–	+	transient	–	nonspec.	–	–	–
Post-traumatic compression	½ or 1	+ or –	if coning	+	+	c.n.3 ½ paresis	nonspec. usually lateralizing	often skull fracture + pineal shift	L.P. dangerous	extra- or subdural haematoma
Pressor reaction	1	–	–	+	–	–	nonspec.	–	–	–
Systemic infections	½ or 1	+ or –	+ or –	+	+ or –	–	nonspec.	–	–	–
Sinusitis	½	–	–	+ or –	–	local tenderness	–	opaque sinuses	–	–
Optic neuritis	½	–	–	–	–	blindness	–	–	–	–
Glaucoma	½	–	–	–	–	raised intraocular tension	–	–	–	–
ACUTE RECURRENT EPISODES										
Subarachnoid haem. (esp. angioma)	1	+	+	+	+	cer. or cerebellar	occ. focal	–	blood-stained	aneurysm angioma
Cerebral vascular insufficiency	½ or 1	–	–	+	–	cer. or b.s.	nonspec.	–	–	vascular stenosis
Intermittent hydrocephalus	1	–	+ or –	+	+ or –	nonspec.	nonspec.	–	–	dilated ventricles

Phaeochromocytoma	1	–	–	+	–	–	nonspec.	–	–	–
Tic Douloureux	½	–	–	–	–	–	–	–	–	–
Cluster	½	+	–	–	–	lacrimation; blocked nostril etc.	–	–	–	–
Migraine	½ or 1	+	+ or –	+ or –	–	cer. or b.s.	normal or nonspec.	–	–	–
SUBACUTE (days or weeks)										
Subdural haematoma	½ or 1	–	if coning	+ or –	+	– or c.n. 3 ½ paresis	lateralizing	pineal shift	L.P. dangerous	localized
Tumour	½ or 1	–	if coning	+ or –	+ or –	cer. or cerebellar	usually focal	pineal shift	L.P. dangerous	localized
Intracranial abscess	½ or 1	–	+ or –	+ or –	+	cer. or cerebellar	focal	pineal shift	L.P. dangerous p.m.n. and lymphocytic usually	localized
Otitic hydrocephalus	1	–	+ or –	+ or –	+ or –	c.n.6 otitis media	nonspec.	mastoiditis	–	normal or small ventricles
Benign intracranial hypertension	1	+ or –	+ or –	+ or –	+ or –	–	nonspec.	–	–	normal or small ventricles
Temporal arteritis	½ or 1	–	–	–	–	scalp vessels; occ. blindness	–	–	–	–
CHRONIC (months or years)										
Tumour	½ or 1	–	if coning	+ or –	+ or –	cer. or b.s.	normal or focal	pineal shift	L.P. dangerous	localized
Eye strain	1	–	–	–	–	refractive errors; heterophoria	–	–	–	–
Bite imbalance	½	–	–	–	–	dental	–	–	–	–
Cervical spondylosis	½ or 1	–	+ or –	+ or –	+ or –	neck crepitus etc.	–	–	–	–
Psychiatric states	1 > ½	mild	–	–	–	–	–	–	–	–
Tension headache	1 > ½	mild	–	–	–	–	–	–	–	–

½ = hemicranial 1 = bilateral headache cer. = cerebral b.s. = brainstem.

Isotope ventriculography

Isotope inserted by lumbar puncture into the CSF usually passes over the hemispheres in the subarachnoid space and is absorbed directly into the superior sagittal sinus. The presence of isotope in the ventricles more than 48 hours after insertion indicates a communicating hydrocephalus or 'normal pressure hydrocephalus'.

Computerized axial tomography (CT scan)

The CT head-scanner uses a focused x-ray beam and detector system to determine the amount of transmitted radiation in each plane traversed by the x-ray beam. The data are analysed by computer and used to

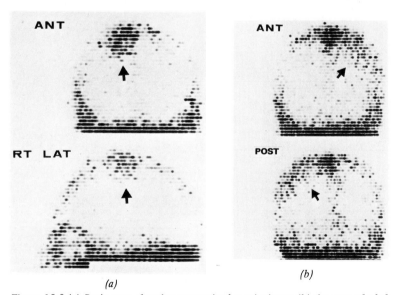

Figure 15.3.(a) Brain scan showing parasagittal meningioma; (b) the scan of a left subdural haematoma or hygroma

construct a cross-sectional radiographic picture of the brain in a number of planes. The CT scan discriminates between density of soft tissue so that a clear picture can be obtained of the cerebral ventricles and sulci. In some instances grey and white matter can be distinguished. The amount of radiation to which the patient is exposed is approximately the same as that of a carotid angiogram.

The patient must remain still during CT scanning so that sedation is required for confused patients. Children may require a general anaesthetic. An intravenous injection of contrast material is required in any patient with a suspected tumour or vascular lesion so that iodine sensitivity should be enquired after and noted on the request form.

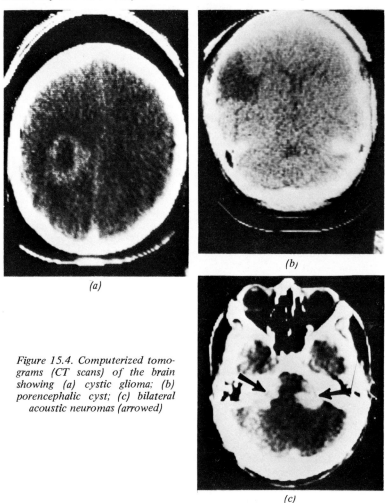

(a)

(b)

(c)

Figure 15.4. Computerized tomograms (CT scans) of the brain showing (a) cystic glioma; (b) porencephalic cyst; (c) bilateral acoustic neuromas (arrowed)

The CT scan is the procedure of choice for demonstrating cerebral atrophy, hydrocephalus or cystic lesions (*Figures 15.4a, b*). It has about the same rate of success in showing tumour or abscess as isotope scanning but will pick up avascular lesions and those which are obscured by anatomical structures in the isotope scan. It can demonstrate acute extradural or subdural haematomas *(Figure 15.4c)* which the isotope scan will not, but is less effective if the haematoma is of more than a few days duration as the density of the haematoma then approaches that of the adjacent cerebral tissue. Isotope scanning therefore remains the procedure of choice for screening for cerebral tumour in cases of headache of recent onset, and the CT scan should be reserved for those in whom suspicion of tumour remains high in spite of a negative isotope scan.

Choice between radionuclide scan and CT scan

Conditions in which a radionuclide scan is likely to be informative

1. Recent onset of epilepsy or headache, suggestive of a space-occupying lesion.
2. Possible cerebral metastases.
3. Cerebral ischaemia.
4. Arteriovenous malformation.
5. Chronic subdural haematoma.

Conditions in which a CT study is likely to be more informative

1. *As initial investigation*
   (a) Suspected obstruction to CSF pathways, hydrocephalus.
   (b) Suspected space-occupying lesion with significant neurological deficit.
   (c) Recent trauma, to exclude acute extradural or subdural haematoma.

2. *Following radionuclide scan*
   (a) Isotope study indicative of space-occupying lesion.
   (b) Elucidation of non-specific scan abnormality, which could be a space-occupying lesion, angioma or cerebral infarction.
   (c) Equivocal result such as an abnormality seen in a single view.
   (d) Negative scan but clinical features suggestive of space-occupying lesion.

Angiography

Cerebral angiography is the only method of demonstrating small cerebral aneurysms and the most specific method for cerebral angiomas. It can be used to determine the blood supply of a tumour that has been picked up by isotope or CT scanning and to outline a subdural haematoma or cerebral abscess. Four-vessel angiography is the only way to demonstrate precisely the site and extent of stenosis of the carotid or vertebral vessels in patients with transient ischaemic attacks. Possible benefit must be weighed against the chances of precipitating cerebral thrombosis in such patients (approximately 2 per cent).

Pneumo-encephalography (PEG)

A PEG is an unpleasant and painful procedure. It may still be required to show up lesions of the posterior fossa or determine the site of obstruction to the CSF pathways, but its traditional role has largely been replaced by CT scanning.

The value of cerebral angiography and air encephalography in the investigation of headache was placed in perspective in a review of the subject by the late Dr Graeme Robertson (1972).

CONCLUSIONS

General practitioners have stated to the author their opinion that diagnosis is easy for neurologists because they have so many investigations at their command. His reply is that special investigations are used sparingly in a minority of patients to confirm or deny a specific hypothesis. If a clinical opinion is firmly based it may stand in spite of negative investigations. We all know of patients who were eventually proven to have a cerebral glioma in spite of investigations repeated at intervals of several years with negative results.

Some of the points which contribute to the diagnosis of headache are set out in Table 15.1, which of necessity oversimplifies the clinical problems, but may be of some assistance in clarifying thoughts on a patient presenting with headache. The more time spent in taking the history of a patient with headache, the more likely are the correct diagnosis and solution to emerge, and the more interesting will the patient's problem appear to the doctor.

One patient was referred to the neurological clinic because of curious episodes of blurred vision, vertigo, dysarthria, ataxia, paraesthesiae and occipital headache, for which he had been investigated thoroughly at enormous expense elsewhere. He had accumulated an impressive dossier which he displayed with a mixture of pride and irritation, since no diagnosis had been reached and his attacks continued. The history disclosed one point that had been missed previously — each attack had been preceded by rapid regular palpitations of the heart. Once his paroxysmal tachycardia was controlled, his episodes of vertebrobasilar insufficiency disappeared.

Complex investigations are no substitute for the time and thought of the physician.

REFERENCES

Goldensohn, E.S. (1976). Paroxysmal and other features of the electroencephalogram in migraine. *Res. clin. Stud. Headache* **4**, 118
Robertson, E.G. (1972). The investigation of headache. *Res. clin. Stud. Headache* **3**, 1
Slatter, K.H. (1968). Some clinical and EEG findings in patients with migraine. *Brain* **91**, 85

Index